Understanding Clinical Research

Understanding
Clinical Research

an introduction

Kathryn Biddle, MA, MB BChir, MRCP
Academic Clinical Fellow at St George's, University of London

Anna Blundell, MSci
Research Assistant in Rheumatology, St George's, University of London

Nidhi Sofat, BSc, MBBS, PhD, FRCP, PGCert, FHEA
Professor of Rheumatology, St George's, University of London
Consultant Rheumatologist, St George's University Hospitals NHS Trust
George's Academic Training (GAT) Lead
Co-Director, PGCert in Research Skills and Methods

Scion

© **Scion Publishing Ltd, 2023**

First published 2023

A CIP catalogue record for this book is available from the British Library.

ISBN 9781914961267

Scion Publishing Limited

The Old Hayloft, Vantage Business Park, Bloxham Road, Banbury OX16 9UX, UK

www.scionpublishing.com

Important Note from the Publisher

The information contained within this book was obtained by Scion Publishing Ltd from sources believed by us to be reliable. However, while every effort has been made to ensure its accuracy, no responsibility for loss or injury whatsoever occasioned to any person acting or refraining from action as a result of information contained herein can be accepted by the authors or publishers.

Readers are reminded that medicine is a constantly evolving science and while the authors and publishers have ensured that all dosages, applications and practices are based on current indications, there may be specific practices which differ between communities. You should always follow the guidelines laid down by the manufacturers of specific products and the relevant authorities in the country in which you are practising.

Although every effort has been made to ensure that all owners of copyright material have been acknowledged in this publication, we would be pleased to acknowledge in subsequent reprints or editions any omissions brought to our attention.

Registered names, trademarks, etc. used in this book, even when not marked as such, are not to be considered unprotected by law.

Cover design by Andrew Magee Design
Typeset by Evolution Design & Digital Ltd (Kent)
Printed in the UK
Last digit is the print number: 10 9 8 7 6 5 4 3 2 1

Contents

Chapter 1   Getting started in clinical research   1

Chapter 2   Designing and appraising clinical studies   9

Foreword

It gives me great pleasure to introduce this important book written by colleagues who exemplify what is achievable in a successful clinical academic career. For medical graduates starting out today, it can be daunting to establish where to start and how to successfully combine medical training with academic activity. Although there are many research opportunities available to those early in their career, it is important for each individual to investigate which specific areas interest them and what skills they will need to develop their research career. This book breaks down the many considerations to support your decision-making and support successfully undertaking research. These include how to get started, how to design and appraise clinical studies, understanding statistical tools needed for specific research questions, ethical considerations, public and patient involvement, qualitative research and the vital dissemination of research findings.

I remain completely convinced that academic activities, alongside clinical practice, are a great route to sustain a long, varied and interesting career. Although at times it may feel daunting, or more complicated, the extra effort is so worth it. This book segments areas of knowledge and demonstrates how things have developed – in research techniques and more broadly. The focus on ethics; the importance of involvement of public and patients in research – not as people to be 'done to' but fully involved in co-designing research areas and outcomes that are important and relevant to them – is welcome.

Of course, clinical academic activity is much broader than conducting research projects and as your experiences develop, you may well focus on a variety of areas, all of which should help your progression. There are contributions to education, knowledge exchange, enterprise; other areas of leadership and citizenship, which may become relevant and allow flexibility in your personal academic pathway. My own career has been very varied and leant on different aspects of academic activity over the years, but cumulatively has helped my progression to a leadership level I could never have imagined at the point of my graduation from medical school. So, be ambitious and go for it in your own way!

Professor Jenny Higham
Vice-Chancellor
St George's, University of London

Preface

Over the last few years clinical research has been a crucial driving force behind significant developments in new treatments in medicine, surgery and primary care. Whilst welcoming these advances in treatments and practice, clinicians and researchers may not always be equipped to assess studies and their methodologies in busy clinical or research environments. This book is aimed at budding researchers who are starting out in research and require further information on the established principles of clinical research. It will also be of interest to the practising clinician and researcher who needs to appraise and consider these developments in evaluating best practice.

There are seven chapters in the book, which cover key topics in initiating research, obtaining funding, design, planning and carrying out of research projects. We also summarise case histories, providing information about how recent medical and science graduates can identify research areas they are interested in. There are chapters on designing and appraising clinical studies, and on types of study, such as expert opinion, case reports, cross-sectional studies, case–control, cohort studies, randomised controlled trials, systematic reviews and meta-analysis. There are also chapters on statistics, data acquisition, analysis and research methodology. A chapter dedicated to ethical considerations and governance is also provided. There is a chapter on qualitative research, mixed methods study design and a dedicated chapter on public and patient involvement, which are important considerations for many studies. The final chapter discusses presenting data as oral or abstract presentations, considerations for publishing and selecting appropriate journals for scientific research.

This book is designed to provide an introduction to clinical research. We focus on the 'why' and the 'how' and discuss the rationale for developing clinical research studies based on the questions that a researcher wants to ask. With the recent Covid-19 worldwide pandemic, many clinicians and researchers were asked to contribute to clinical studies and trials which led to the rapid development of new therapies and vaccines for combating the pandemic. Such an international effort required rapid upskilling by the workforce to equip them with the skills required in conducting and reporting clinical research in a time-restricted environment. Many of the published studies for Covid-19 are used as case histories in the book, with worked examples on the types of study, statistical analyses and reporting outcomes. Our examples demonstrate how evidence-based practice is developed through research.

Our book embodies the Postgraduate Certificate in Research Skills and Methods curriculum at St George's, University of London and can also be used as an accompanying text for other PGCert and Masters courses in clinical research. It will also be helpful to those who are embarking on MD/PhD studies.

Kathryn Biddle
Anna Blundell
Nidhi Sofat

Acknowledgements

The authors would like to thank Dr Mathew John Paul for useful discussions and Ms Yvonne Forde for her support in proofreading.

We would also like to thank all our families for their patience and support during the writing of this book – we couldn't have done it without you!

About the authors

Dr Kathryn Biddle trained in Medicine at the University of Cambridge. Following her Foundation year training, she was awarded an Academic Clinical Fellowship from the NIHR (National Institute for Health and Care Research) which allowed her to continue her clinical training in Rheumatology combined with training in academic research. Kathryn is continuing her training as a Clinical Academic.

Anna Blundell completed her Master in Science degree at the University of Bath. Following this she worked as a Research Assistant on clinical trials and translational studies at St George's, University of London. She is currently pursuing her PhD studies.

Professor Nidhi Sofat studied Medicine at University College London. She then trained in Rheumatology at Imperial College Healthcare NHS Trust and was awarded her PhD at the Kennedy Institute for Rheumatology, funded by a Clinical Research Training Fellowship from the Wellcome Trust. Nidhi works as a Consultant Rheumatologist at St George's University Hospitals and also leads her own research group in Translational Medicine at St George's, University of London, where she is the National Institute for Health and Care Research (NIHR) Integrated Academic Training programme lead for Clinical Academic trainees.

Abbreviations

ACF	Academic Clinical Fellow
AE	adverse event
AR	adverse reaction
ARR	absolute risk reduction
AUC	area under the curve
BHF	British Heart Foundation
CAQDAS	computer-assisted qualitative data analysis software
CCT	Certificate of Completion of Training
CI	confidence interval; chief investigator
CRF	case report form
CTIMP	clinical trial of an IMP
df	degrees of freedom
EBM	evidence-based medicine
GCP	Good Clinical Practice
HR	hazard ratio
HRA	Health Research Authority
IMP	investigational medicinal product
IQR	interquartile range
IRAS	Integrated Research Application System
ISF	investigator site file
LR	likelihood ratio
MHRA	Medicines and Healthcare products Regulatory Agency
MRC	Medical Research Council
NIHR	National Institute for Health and Care Research
NNT	number needed to treat
NPV	negative predictive value
OR	odds ratio
PI	principal investigator
PiiAF	Public Involvement Impact Assessment
PIL	patient information leaflet
PPI	public and patient involvement
PPV	positive predictive value
RCT	randomised controlled trial
REC	research ethics committee
ROC	receiver operating characteristic
RR	relative risk
RSI	Reference Safety Information
SAE	serious adverse event
SD	standard deviation
SEM	standard error of the mean
SFP	Specialised Foundation Programme

CHAPTER 1

Getting started in clinical research

1.1 Introduction

Getting started in research can be challenging as there is a lot of information out there. A good starting point might be one of your lecturers from university or reading recent papers on a topic that you are interested in. What inspires you? It is important to find out what you like and also what you may not like so much. It may be possible to organise taster sessions with a research group, shadow a team involved in clinical trials and also access resources that are widely available online, e.g. online resources from the NIHR Academy (www.nihr.ac.uk/explore-nihr/support/academy.htm), UK Research and Innovation (www.ukri.org) and the Wellcome Trust (https://wellcome.org/grant-funding). Funding bodies publish information about their schemes and what previously funded students and trainees have done, e.g. The Wellcome Trust, the National Institute for Health and Care Research (NIHR), the Medical Research Council (MRC) and the British Heart Foundation (BHF). Such resources are an invaluable source of information and further information is provided in *Section 1.9*.

1.2 What types of research are there?

There are many types of research and it is important to find out as much as you can about what you are interested in before you decide on an area that you want to work in. Many universities and hospitals now offer taster days which allow trainees to gain some experience of how projects run in their unit, which can provide a gentle introduction to a subject and to see if it is of interest. Early experience may also help the trainee work out which area they are interested in working in.

1.2.1 Laboratory-based research

Laboratory-based research often focuses on the study of molecular pathways and mediators that form part of fundamental processes in physiology and cell biology. Changes in these pathways during pathology are often studied, with a focus on a key protein and/or molecular mediators of a process or pathway that could offer options for treatment, e.g. a protein inhibitor.

Some medical students may have done a laboratory-based project during medical school and enjoyed the work they have done. This could then continue beyond medical school with work towards a higher degree, e.g. PhD. Many of these projects are asking fundamental science-based questions. Ask yourself if a few years working in a laboratory appeals to you and whether you enjoy the practical side of doing experiments. Ask yourself if you like trouble-shooting with assays, because there will be times when things are not working and you have to try to establish solutions. But at the end of the project, you might have discovered a new pathway or a new compound that may hold promise in treating a specific condition.

1.2.2 Clinical studies and clinical trials

Clinical studies and clinical trials form the cornerstone of biomedical research. Often, a compound which has been tested in the laboratory shows potential in the treatment of a particular condition and is ready for testing in clinical studies. These studies may take different forms, depending on the phase of the compound in its drug development. For example, a phase 1 study would be performed to test a drug for the first time in humans, a phase 2 study could be conducted to test in people with a particular condition, a phase 3 study would be a large randomised controlled trial (often placebo-controlled), and a phase 4 study would include post-marketing surveillance of a drug after licensing.

Other clinical studies may include observational studies, e.g. cohort studies of subjects with a particular condition such as cardiovascular disease or diabetes mellitus over time.

Some trainees may enjoy clinical science more and want to get involved with patient assessments and clinical outcome measures. Taster days are available in clinical trial units or clinical research facilities, which can provide excellent information on how to run clinical studies and the day-to-day experience of what is involved. There is a high demand for well-conducted clinical studies, therefore there is a high demand for appropriately qualified medical practitioners who can conduct clinical research.

1.2.3 Epidemiological studies

Population health studies with large datasets are also an option for those interested in big data, and epidemiological research covers a wide range of approaches and scientific themes, e.g. population health, cardiovascular disease, and population genetics using genome-wide association studies.

The different stages at which you can get involved in research during your medical training are summarised in *Figure 1.1*.

Opportunities for research exist at all stages of training, from the undergraduate level through to core and specialist training. An interest in research may begin with a special study module (SSM) or intercalated BSc project during medical school training, followed by research projects during foundation year and specialist training. Conducting research during clinical training can be potentiated by dedicated academic training programmes which allow the completion of both clinical and academic research

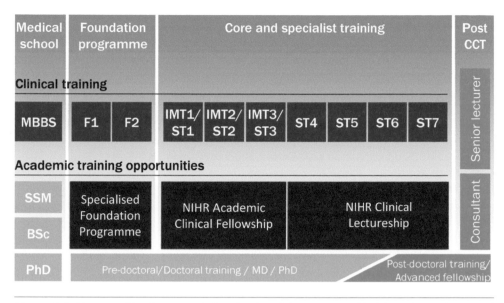

Medical school	Foundation programme	Core and specialist training							Post CCT

Clinical training

MBBS	F1	F2	IMT1/ ST1	IMT2/ ST2	IMT3/ ST3	ST4	ST5	ST6	ST7	Senior lecturer

Academic training opportunities

SSM	Specialised Foundation Programme	NIHR Academic Clinical Fellowship	NIHR Clinical Lectureship	Consultant
BSc				
PhD	Pre-doctoral/Doctoral training / MD / PhD		Post-doctoral training/ Advanced fellowship	

Figure 1.1. Opportunities for research (academic training opportunities) in undergraduate and graduate medical training.

training, such as the NIHR-funded Academic Foundation Training Programme and Academic Clinical Fellowships.

1.3 How to get involved as a medical student

As described above, there are several ways of gaining exposure to research during undergraduate medicine. These include doing intercalated BSc projects in your chosen field of interest, special study modules and also elective projects. You may be able to choose several projects which then help you to build up a portfolio, e.g. if you are interested in public health, you may want to look at vaccination rates for Covid-19 in a specific area and the reasons for people not taking up the vaccine. This could be followed up by an elective project assisting with vaccination programmes abroad. Building a personalised portfolio will help you develop your career interests and combine research with clinical work and training.

1.4 How to get involved as a trainee

Most medical graduates in the UK complete their medical training and pursue higher research degrees once they have chosen their specialism, e.g. surgery, medicine, primary care. There are then several pathways that can be followed (*Figure 1.1*).

The NIHR Integrated Academic Training programme is a national scheme which allows trainees to pursue dedicated research training alongside their clinical training. Progressing through the programme is contingent on achieving clinical competencies. Typically, for trainees qualifying after medical school and pursuing the Specialised Foundation Programme (SFP), they will be able to do research projects for 4 months out of their total 2-year block. For Academic Clinical Fellows (ACFs), there is the opportunity to conduct 9 months of research in their chosen area out of a total of 3 years of training; the research can be undertaken during core training or specialist training. The aim is to develop a basic understanding of research skills and conduct some preliminary work towards an application for a PhD Fellowship; this is a competitive application process through various funding bodies which may be relevant to the applicant's research area, e.g. British Heart Foundation, NIHR, the Wellcome Trust and other charities. Many candidates complete a Postgraduate Diploma in Research Skills and Methods during their SFP or ACF so that they acquire the skills needed to pursue further research in their area of interest.

1.5   Deciding which higher degree to undertake

It can often be difficult to decide which research degree to undertake. Some candidates plan to spend a shorter amount of time out of their clinical training and may choose to pursue a Masters (MSc) or MD(Res) which provides focused and dedicated research training in a specific area. Other candidates may plan to pursue a longer research period and apply for a PhD fellowship award, providing them with 3 years of funding to pursue their PhD. It is generally acknowledged that if a candidate is interested in pursuing an academic career, then undertaking a PhD is more desirable, to develop the rigour of academic research, and it is likely to benefit the trainee as they progress through their career.

1.6   Funding considerations

Applying for and being awarded PhD funding is often a long process. It takes time to formulate a proposal that will be considered appropriate for external funding. It is important to identify the person, the project and the place where you will pursue your research. For example, can you assemble an excellent supervisory team who will support you through your PhD and help you achieve your objectives? Is there a leader in the field that you can identify and discuss your ideas with? Who else do you need to work with? Do you need to identify a clinical trials unit and a statistician?

Some trainees may have an interest in a particular disease area and can apply for relevant positions through university schemes that advertise clinical PhD fellowships through their websites. Other organisations, such as the Francis Crick Institute in London and other large biomedical research centres, have their own PhD schemes which trainees can apply to. Other schemes which allow applications every year for clinical fellowships include the NIHR, MRC, BHF and the Wellcome Trust.

If you have your own specific ideas as to the area you want to study, then you'll need to assemble a team who can assist you in developing your project, protocols and grant proposal. Once you identify a potential supervisor and university you want to work in, you will be provided with assistance to develop your objectives. It is important to find out early about which funding bodies are interested in supporting your research area. For example, if you have a clinical project which involves conducting clinical trials, you may want to apply to NIHR; in contrast, if you are working on a more fundamental lab-based science project, the MRC, BHF or the Wellcome Trust may be more likely to fund your work. There can be up to 6–9 months between applications being submitted and hearing about interviews or awards, so it is important to plan ahead, including costing your project in detail for salary, consumables and other costs.

Once you have been awarded funding, you will also need to discuss your plans with the Training Programme Director for your specialty because you are likely to need to take time out of your clinical rotation to gain your Out of Programme Research (OOPR) during your PhD studies.

1.7 Case histories

Below are a series of case histories from trainees who combined academic research with clinical careers. The summaries help to highlight the varied paths that are possible in developing an academic career.

Case history 1

AM qualified in Medicine from the University of Cambridge. As a trainee, he was interested in pursuing a career in cardiology. After his foundation year and core medical training in Cambridge, he joined a cardiology rotation in the Oxford region. It was during his specialist training that he became interested in research and so he approached several potential supervisors, in both London and the Oxford region. He decided to pursue a PhD in London focused on cardiological factors influencing sudden death in athletes and also worked with the Football Association on collecting data. Working with his supervisory team, he was able to analyse and present his data at national and international meetings and was able to publish his work in the *New England Journal of Medicine*. After gaining his PhD, he applied for an NIHR Clinical Lecturer post in the same unit in London where he undertook his research. He continued to develop his skills in assessing athletes at risk of sudden death. After completing his clinical lectureship, and being awarded his CCT (Certificate of Completion of Training), he was recruited to a Clinical Senior Lecturer and Honorary Consultant in Cardiology position in Manchester.

This case history demonstrates how it is possible to develop a research interest in a chosen field and acquire skills that may be unique to a particular area. The skills acquired were then applied to develop a programme of work that AM implemented in a new unit where he was appointed to a substantive position.

Case history 2

DB qualified in Medicine from University College London. As a trainee, he became interested in Pharmacology and successfully applied for an NIHR Academic Clinical Fellowship in London. The position provided DB with 9 months of protected research time over a 3-year training period, which helped him to develop his research interests. He then applied for an NIHR Doctoral Research Training Fellowship in COPD-related research, which he was awarded. He completed his PhD and was also awarded a PGCert in Medical Education. During his period as a clinical pharmacology trainee, he was also a visiting scientist at GlaxoSmithKline as a project physician in discovery medicine, he co-authored a pharmacology textbook and joined the *British National Formulary* Joint Formulary Committee.

DB applied for a substantive position in London and is currently a Consultant Physician in General Internal Medicine and Clinical Pharmacology. He is also an Honorary Clinical Lecturer and maintains his teaching portfolio.

This example shows how DB was able to start his academic career through the NIHR ACF scheme and then go on to a PhD via the NIHR Doctoral Research Training Fellowship. He was subsequently offered a substantive Consultant post after completing his training and has been able to continue his research and teaching interests.

Case history 3

KS qualified in Medicine from the University of Oxford and she was interested in becoming a Consultant in vascular surgery. She did not initially plan to be an academic surgeon, but reconciled herself to the fact that she would need to undertake a higher degree in order to be competitive at interview. She had some friends who'd successfully completed MD(Res) and PhDs. She applied to do an MD(Res) at a vascular research institute in London, studying a new treatment for abdominal aortic aneurysm repair. She thoroughly enjoyed the research and was able to present her findings at national and international meetings before qualifying. KS then applied for an NIHR-funded clinical lectureship in which she continued the work that she developed during her MD(Res); she also developed her teaching and supervision skills. KS has subsequently been awarded her CCT and is now a post-CCT Fellow in Vascular Surgery. She plans to continue to a substantive Consultant position and maintain her interest in research and teaching.

The example of KS shows how it is possible to pursue academic interests later on in training. It also demonstrates that it is possible to pursue academic interests in surgery, which is often perceived as a challenging field in which to research. KS was able to combine local funding and NIHR-backed opportunities to pursue her academic research.

1.8   Chapter summary

This opening chapter has highlighted the multitude of opportunities an academic career can bring. However, it is not an easy path to navigate and requires careful planning, aptitude and commitment.

Being awarded your research degree marks a milestone and indicates that you have successfully undertaken novel research, which has been examined independently.

After their period of research, many trainees will go back into clinical training and will subsequently pursue clinical careers, but they may maintain an interest in research; for example, by becoming a Principal Investigator for a clinical trial. Others may want to continue research and will aim to combine it with a clinical career. There is a well-established clinical academic career pathway for this, with similar recognition to non-clinical academics, e.g. progressing from Senior Lecturer to Professor.

1.9   References and useful websites

The Academy of Medical Sciences: https://acmedsci.ac.uk

The Gold Guide, 8th edition – Conference of Postgraduate Medical Deans: www.copmed.org.uk/gold-guide/gold-guide-8th-edition

NIHR: www.nihr.ac.uk/explore-nihr/academy-programmes/integrated-academic-training.htm

UK Research and Innovation: www.ukri.org/opportunity/clinical-research-training-fellowship

Wellcome Trust: https://wellcome.org/grant-funding/schemes/phd-fellowships-health-professionals

02

Designing and appraising clinical studies

2.1 Introduction

One of the most important considerations in designing a clinical study is the research question. In order to synthesise pertinent new research questions, it is important to review and appraise the existing literature in the field.

Considerations and points for literature review include:

- Are there any randomised trials that have already been done in the area?
  - What are the results from these trials? Are there areas of outstanding uncertainty?
  - What is the quality of these trials? Can the existing evidence be trusted?
- Is there a need for a new study?
  - If high quality data already exists, there is little point in repeating a study.
- Would it be more useful to do a meta-analysis from published trials?
  - This may be the case when multiple randomised controlled trials have been performed but a consensus has yet to be reached. If there are not enough clinical trials in a research area that can be subjected to meta-analysis, then a systematic review may be more appropriate.

Following literature review, an appropriate study design must be chosen to answer the research question. In this chapter, we will discuss the development and appraisal of different study types.

2.2 What kinds of study are there?

Different study designs are used to answer different clinical questions. The variety of study designs is outlined in the evidence pyramid which is depicted below (*Fig. 2.1*). As we go from the bottom of the pyramid to the top, studies have increasing quality of evidence and are considered to be more robust.

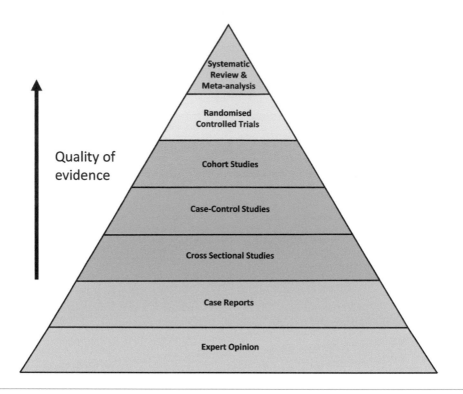

Figure 2.1. The hierarchy of different types of clinical studies. The methodologies associated with each type of study are distinct. As one travels up the pyramid, the quality of evidence is increased.

This chapter will take you through the various types of study, from the bottom of the pyramid to the top. By working through examples of each study, we will discuss the relevant applications, benefits and downsides.

2.3   General considerations in clinical research

All studies are liable to error including bias and confounding. These factors must be considered in the planning and appraisal of all types of clinical study.

2.3.1 Identifying and minimising sources of bias

Bias describes systematic error in the design or the conduct of a clinical trial that encourages one outcome over the other. Bias affects the **validity** of clinical research and explains why some clinical studies result in incorrect conclusions.

Bias can occur at any stage of study design from planning to publication. Whilst studies at the top of the pyramid of evidence are at least risk, all studies are liable to bias. The common types of bias differ between different studies and this will be discussed in more detail in the relevant sections of this chapter.

2.3.2 Consideration of confounding

Confounding is an important source of bias. It occurs when an external factor is associated with both the exposure and the outcome of interest. **The presence of confounding means that correlation does not imply causation** (see *Fig. 2.2*). This is very important to remember! Although research studies can show us whether two factors are associated with each other, this does not mean that one causes the other. For example, imagine an observational study where participants were given a mental health questionnaire and asked how long they slept each night. If this study found an association between oversleeping and depression, this does not necessarily mean that oversleeping causes depression. Alternatively, depression may cause oversleeping; this is known as **reverse causality**. Moreover, there may be other variables at play which affect both sleep and depression. For example, oversleeping may be associated with unemployment or poor physical health which in turn may be associated with depression. In this example, unemployment and poor health are possible **confounding** variables. They are defined as factors that influence both the dependent and the independent variables, hence affecting the measured association between the two factors. It is important to consider the influence of confounding factors in all studies in order to avoid making erroneous conclusions. Different methods for avoiding the effects of confounding are used in different studies.

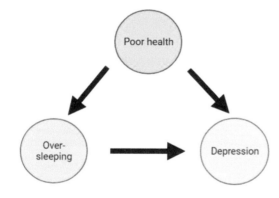

Figure 2.2. In this example, poor health influences depression and over-sleeping and therefore acts as a confounding variable.

2.4 Expert opinion

Opinion articles report information from key leaders in the field on new developments in treatment or diagnosis. They can provide a useful insight, but are often biased by the author's opinions and previous experience. This evidence is not considered rigorous.

2.5 Case reports and case series

Case reports describe the clinical presentation, investigation results, treatment and follow-up of an individual patient. Most commonly, they report an unusual or novel presentation, condition or response to therapy. As such, they remain an important form of communication within the medical literature. For example, they can provide insight into rare conditions, highlight novel pathologies and can be an important first step in the recognition of a trend. As they are relatively easy to write and read, they can be an attractive form of research to conduct and publish by busy clinicians. Although they can highlight useful learning points and guide areas of future research, their interpretation is limited by the effects of bias or chance and it is clear that individual cases cannot guide population-wide clinical guidelines.

Case series refer to the report of more than one clinical case. Most of these studies are retrospective and share the same characteristics and limitations to case reports. Therefore, these studies require replication in larger datasets to confirm the association and direct further clinical management.

2.6   A summary of observational studies

The next part of the chapter will focus on the three main types of observational studies including cross-sectional studies, case-control studies and cohort studies.

Observational studies usually measure the association between an exposure (**independent variable**) and outcome (**dependent variable**). In observational studies, researchers do not intervene; this means that they simply measure the effect of an exposure without manipulating conditions, i.e. subjects are permitted to continue as they would without being in a clinical trial. They can be described as prospective where participants are monitored over time, or retrospective where information is collected about the past. Observational studies contrast to experimental studies such as randomised controlled trials (RCTs) where the researcher measures the effects of an intervention in a controlled setting. Although RCTs are the best way to determine causality between variables, there are many cases in which observational studies are more appropriate:

1. **It would not be ethical to conduct a randomised controlled trial.** For example, a RCT investigating the association between alcohol intake and the development of liver disease would entail the randomisation of participants to groups with different levels of alcohol intake. Obviously, it would not be ethical for a researcher to make this intervention and observational study methods, such as cohort studies, are required to characterise this particular association.

2. **A rare event is being studied.** It would be resource-intensive to conduct a controlled trial for a very long time period to see if a rare event occurs following an intervention. Observational studies are often preferable when studying rare events, as retrospective analysis can be performed after the event has occurred.

3. **To generate hypotheses to test in an experimental study.** RCTs are expensive and time-consuming. Therefore, conducting initial observational studies can be a good starting point before carrying out experimental studies.

2.6.1 **Sources of bias in observational studies**

Observational studies are prone to certain types of bias. Common types of bias to consider include:

Selection bias

Selection bias occurs when the study sample is not representative of the general population. In clinical research, cultural, language and social barriers may hinder participation from certain groups. These barriers often limit the generalisability of the results to wider populations (also known as the external validity of the study).

Selection bias is a common problem in all research studies. Participants who volunteer to participate in research may be systematically different from those who do not. For example, in an observational study investigating the association between activity levels and heart disease, sedentary individuals may be unlikely to participate due to embarrassment or fear of judgement.

Certain types of sampling methods are more prone to bias; this will be discussed in more detail in *Section 3.2.2*.

Reporting or recall bias

Observational studies are prone to reporting or **recall bias**. Reporting bias occurs when participants knowingly or unknowingly report inaccurate data. This is a common problem in studies involving the use of questionnaires. Recall bias is a particular issue in retrospective observational studies. This occurs when participants incorrectly report exposures in the past.

Attrition bias

Attrition bias occurs in studies that follow participants over a period of time. It describes when participants drop out of the study and do not complete follow-up. When these participants are systematically different to participants who complete the study, attrition bias impacts study validity and introduces a source of error into the results.

2.7 **Cross-sectional studies**

Cross-sectional studies are observational studies that measure the frequency of exposure and outcome in study participants at a specific point in time. Cross-sectional studies report in terms of prevalence, where prevalence is defined as the proportion of a population who have a specific characteristic at a given time-point. Several methods are used to report prevalence:

- **Point prevalence**: the proportion of a population who have the characteristic at a specific point in time

- **Period prevalence**: the proportion of a population who have the characteristic at any point over the pre-specified time period
- **Lifetime prevalence**: the proportion of a population who have the characteristic at any point over their entire lifetime.

Cross-sectional studies are commonly used to assess the prevalence of disease in a population and can be used to characterise the association between an exposure and outcome. Advantages of cross-sectional studies are that they are relatively quick, cheap and easy to conduct. Furthermore, they can allow us to look at a large study population and this can be used to generate hypotheses to plan larger cohort studies. Cross-sectional studies are commonly used by public health programmes to monitor healthcare interventions and to plan healthcare policy. For example, a cross-sectional study may measure the prevalence of antibiotic resistance in a hospital population. This information may be used to write microbiology guidelines and inform antibiotic prescribing.

There are several limitations of cross-sectional studies. Since these studies are taking a snapshot in time, it is not possible to derive temporal or causal relationships between exposure and outcome. Furthermore, cross-sectional studies cannot tell us about the number of new cases of disease development over a specified time period (**incidence**). Therefore, cross-sectional studies are not informative in describing patterns of new disease development.

Cross-sectional studies are prone to certain types of bias. The measurements taken at a single time-point may not be representative of the overall association between exposure and outcome. For example, a cross-sectional study which measures the relationship between dietary intake and Body Mass Index (BMI) will result in erroneous conclusions if the overweight participants have commenced a low-calorie diet during the period of data collection. This could lead the researchers to incorrectly conclude that low-calorie intake is associated with increased BMI. Therefore, the results from cross-sectional studies must be interpreted with caution and the influence of bias must be carefully considered.

The worked example below will show you how to plan and appraise a cross-sectional study.

WORKED EXAMPLE
Beer and obesity: a cross-sectional study

Bobak *et al.* (2003) *Eur J Clin Nutr*, 57: 1250; doi.org/10.1038/sj.ejcn.1601678

Study aim
This study aimed to see if the 'beer belly' was a real phenomenon by examining whether beer consumption was related to waist–hip ratio (WHR) and BMI.

Methods
In this study, the researchers used a random sample of 1141 men and 1212 women from the Czech Republic.

Recruited participants completed a questionnaire and underwent an examination to measure BMI and WHR. Subjects were asked to report the frequency of alcohol intake during a typical week and to complete a 24-hour dietary recall. The information gathered from the 24-hour recall was used to assess the reporting of beer intake during a typical week at the group level.

The association between beer intake and BMI and WHR was analysed with linear regression, separating men and women.

Comments

- Using a large sample is important in order to ensure that your study is representative of the population you are investigating.

- A random sampling method means that every individual in the population has an equal chance of being recruited; this helps to reduce selection bias. More information about sampling methods is summarised in *Section 3.2.2*.

- Self-report methods are susceptible to bias, as participants may misremember or not tell the truth. In this study, two self-reporting methods were used to estimate beer intake. Although this increases the reliability of the data, the results are still prone to reporting or recall bias. Other sources of bias include measurement bias, as readings may have been influenced by factors such as time of year or day of the week.

- Linear regression is a type of statistical analysis that models the relationship between a dependent variable and one or more explanatory variables. This is described in more detail in *Section 3.8.3*.

Results
The results from the study are summarised in *Table 2.1*.

891 men and 1098 women were included in the analysis, which only included exclusive beer drinkers and non-drinkers.

Table 2.1: WHR and BMI by weekly beer intake

		WHR		BMI	
	No. of subjects	Age–adjusted	Multivariate*	Age–adjusted	Multivariate*
Men (N=891)					
Nondrinkers	227	0.0 (reference category)	0.0 (reference category)	0.0 (reference category)	0.0 (reference category)
≤1 l/week	145	0.003 (−0.009; 0.016)	0.003 (−0.010; 0.019)	−0.03 (−0.81; 0.75)	0.03 (−0.83; 0.89)
1.1–3.5 l/week	232	0.006 (−0.004; 0.017)	0.004 (−0.008; 0.015)	0.05 (−0.64; 0.74)	0.04 (−0.72; 0.79)
3.6–7 l/week	209	0.014 (0.003; 0.025)	0.008 (−0.004; 0.021)	0.11 (−0.60; 0.82)	0.05 (−0.74; 0.84)
>7 l/week	78	0.021 (0.006; 0.036)	0.010 (−0.006; 0.027)	−0.21 (−1.18; 0.76)	−0.13 (−1.12; 0.95)
Trend (per 1 l/week)		0.0017 (0.0007; 0.0029)	0.0009 (−0.0003; 0.0020)	−0.01 (−0.07; 0.06)	−0.01 (−0.08; 0.07)
P for trend		0.001	0.143	0.831	0.891
Women (N=1098)					
Nondrinkers	917	0.0 (reference category)	0.0 (reference category)	0.0 (reference category)	0.0 (reference category)
≤1 l/week	122	−0.009 (−0.020; 0.002)	−0.007 (−0.01 8; 0.005)	−0.20 (−1.13; 0.73)	0.16 (−0.83; 1.15)
1.1–3.5 l/week	37	−0.002 (−0.020; 0.017)	−0.007 (−0.029; 0.014)	−1.56 (−3. 17; 0.06)	−1.72 (−3.82; 0.05)
>3.5 l/week	22	0.006 (−0.021;0.031)	0.010 (−0.020; 0.040)	−1.88 (−3.95; 0.19)	−1.64 (−3.51; 0.55)
Trend (per 1 l/week)		−0.001 (−0.005;0.004)	0.000 (−0.005; 0.005)	−0.34 (−0.65; −0.03)	−0.26 (−0.60; 0.07)
P for trend		0.813	0.938	0.030	0.098

*Adjusted for age, cigarettes/day physical activity, total cholestrol and education.

Material reproduced from *European Journal of Clinical Nutrition*, 57: 1250, with permission from Springer Nature.

The participants were divided into four groups according to their average weekly intake of beer: non-drinkers; ≤1L; 1.1–3.5L; 3.6–7L; and >7L. The two highest categories were pooled for women. Overall, the mean weekly beer intake was 3.1L in men and 0.3L in women.

The study found that beer intake was positively correlated to WHR in men and negatively correlated to BMI in women. However, after the analysis was adjusted for confounding variables including physical activity, BMI, smoking and education, these correlations lost statistical significance. This data is summarised in *Table 2.1.*

Comments

- People who drank other alcoholic drinks were excluded so that effects from other alcoholic drinks would not confound the results.
- Statistical methods can be used to adjust for the effects of confounding factors. When this was done, there was no correlation between beer intake and WHR/BMI. This highlights the importance of adjusting for confounding to reduce the likelihood of false positive reports.

Conclusion

Overall, the study concluded that beer intake was weakly positively associated with WHR in men and weakly negatively associated with BMI in women. These associations lost statistical significance when analysis was adjusted for confounding factors. This suggests there is no correlation with beer drinking and obesity.

Comments

- In this study, there was no association between beer intake and obesity after confounding factors were adjusted for.
- As this sample consisted mainly of people who drank moderately, the results cannot be generalised to groups who drink heavily. In all clinical studies, care must be taken to ensure that conclusions are not inappropriately applied to populations with different demographic, behavioural or clinical features.

2.8   Case–control studies

Case–control studies are another way to investigate the relationship between an exposure and outcome. In a case–control study, people with a particular outcome, usually a specific disease, are compared to people without. Exposures are factors of interest that may be associated with developing the outcome. In case–control studies, exposures are assessed retrospectively. Case–control studies are particularly useful when investigating the development of rare diseases. They can also be used to measure multiple exposures in a single study design.

As in all studies, it is important that confounding variables are measured and accounted for. To adjust for potential confounders in case–control studies, participants from the control group are matched to participants in the case group. Matching is generally performed on the basis of characteristics such as gender, BMI, age and ethnicity. This is known as a matched-pairs design and aims to ensure an equal distribution of characteristics in both groups. Through matching, the effects of confounding factors are minimised, although they cannot be removed completely.

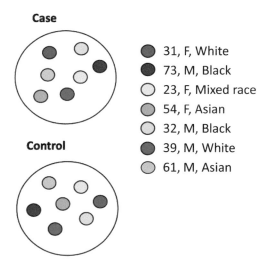

Case

31, F, White
73, M, Black
23, F, Mixed race
54, F, Asian
32, M, Black
39, M, White
61, M, Asian

Control

Figure 2.3. A matched pairs design. In this example, participants have been matched on the basis of age, sex and ethnicity.

2.8.1 Odds ratio

Case–control studies allow us to measure the association between an exposure and an outcome. This is commonly expressed as an odds ratio. The **odds ratio** describes the odds that an outcome will occur given a particular exposure, compared to the odds of the outcome occurring in the absence of the exposure.

The following worked example demonstrates the steps required to calculate an odds ratio using the results from a case–control study.

WORKED EXAMPLE
Benzodiazepine use and risk of Alzheimer's disease: case–control study

This study investigated the association between the use of benzodiazepines and the development of Alzheimer's disease. The results from the study are summarised in *Table 2.2*. In this example, the exposure of interest is benzodiazepine use and the outcome is Alzheimer's disease.

Table 2.2: A 2×2 table outlining the frequencies of benzodiazepine use in those with and without Alzheimer's disease

	Alzheimer's disease	Healthy control
Benzodiazepine use	894 (A)	2873 (B)
No benzodiazepine use	902 (C)	4311 (D)

De Gage *et al.* (2014), *BMJ*, 349: g5205, doi.org/10.1136/bmj.g5205

In this example, the odds ratio can be calculated using the following steps:

Odds ratio (OR) = odds of diseased in exposed / odds of disease in not exposed

= (A/B) / (C/D)

= (894/2873) / (902/4311) = 1.49

This is the same as AD / CB

> ### Comments
>
> In this worked example, the results can be interpreted in the following manner:
>
> *Participants taking benzodiazepines have 1.49 times the odds of developing dementia compared to those who do not take benzodiazepines.*
>
> We cannot conclude that benzodiazepines cause dementia as confounding factors may be at play.
>
> In general, the interpretation of OR is as follows:
>
> - OR >1: more people with the disease were subject to the exposure than people without the disease. This suggests that the exposure is associated with development of the disease.
> - OR = 1: there was an equal frequency of exposure in people with and without the disease. This suggests that there is no association between the exposure and the development of the disease.
> - OR <1: fewer people with the disease were subject to the exposure compared to those without the disease. This suggests that the exposure may exert a protective effect against the development of the disease.
>
> The OR is discussed in more detail in *Section 3.7.1*.

2.8.2 Confidence interval

In case–control studies, a **confidence interval (CI)** is commonly reported alongside the odds ratio. The confidence interval is used to estimate the precision of the odds ratio; a large CI indicates a high level of uncertainty whilst a small CI indicates a higher level of precision. Generally, a confidence level of 95% is reported and this denotes a 95% probability that the true value falls within the stated range. The CI is often used as a proxy for statistical significance. When the CI overlaps the null value (i.e. OR = 1), there is no statistically significant association between the exposure and the outcome. *Section 3.3.3* outlines the steps involved in calculating the CI.

WORKED EXAMPLE
Association between cardiometabolic disease and severe COVID-19: a nationwide case–control study of patients requiring invasive mechanical ventilation

Svensson *et al*. (2021), *BMJ Open*, 11: e044486, doi.org/10.1136/bmjopen-2020-044486

Study aims

This study aimed to find out whether individuals with diabetes, obesity and hypertension were at increased risk of developing severe Covid-19. Therefore, the exposures of interest were diabetes, obesity and hypertension. The outcome of interest was severe Covid-19; this was defined as hospitalisation and requirement for ventilation.

Cases

In this study, severe Covid-19 was defined as laboratory-confirmed SARS-CoV-2 infection in individuals admitted to intensive care unit (ICU) and treated with mechanical ventilation. Eligible patients were identified from the Swedish Intensive Care Registry (SIR). In total, 1086 patients met the inclusion criteria.

> Comments
> - The first step in planning a case–control study is defining a strict set of requirements that constitutes a 'case'. For instance, if the case is a disease, the subtype, severity and diagnostic criteria must be defined.
> - This is an example of well-defined inclusion criteria for identifying eligible cases with severe disease.
> - In this study, all eligible patients were identified on the basis of admission to ICU. In general, defining cases using incidence rates, for example admission rates to ICU, is advantageous over measuring population prevalence, which is also affected by disease duration.

Controls

In this study, for each enrolled case, 10 matched control participants were randomly selected from the Swedish Population Register (10,860 in total). These cases were matched based on age, sex and district of residence.

> **Comments**
> - After defining the inclusion criteria that constitute the 'case', a method for recruiting control participants must be considered. This can be difficult because the control group must be well-matched to the case group. Specifically, the control group must be from the same source population and must also be 'at risk' of developing the disease. For example, the control group for cases of prostate cancer cannot be females.
> - Healthy individuals from the general population are commonly recruited to the control group. These controls are likely to have had similar exposures to the case group. A disadvantage is that they may find it more difficult to recall exposures than the case group, who often have an interest in the cause of their illness. In some cases, controls with other diseases can be selected in an attempt to minimise the effect of recall bias.
> - In some case–control studies, including this example, multiple controls are matched to each case to increase statistical power. This is particularly relevant when the number of cases is small; for example, with rare diseases.
> - Matching for age, sex and district of residence was a method of minimising the effect of confounding variables. For example, increased age and male gender are well-known to increase Covid-19 severity. By ensuring that the two groups are well-matched with regard to age and gender profile, the effects of these confounding variables are minimised.

Matching the cases on the basis of district of residence is important to further reduce confounding factors. As the case and control population come from the same source population, their risk of developing Covid-19 should be similar. Furthermore, the dominant circulating Covid-19 variant should be similar in populations from the same district.

Assessing exposure

In this study, the exposures of interest were obesity, hypertension and type 2 diabetes. A history of the relevant disease was based on recorded diagnosis in the National Patient Register within the preceding 15 years or prescribed drugs within the preceding 12 months. Specifically, the National Patient Register in Sweden recorded a large number of comorbidities including hypertension, hyperlipidaemia, type 2 diabetes mellitus, heart failure and cardiovascular disease (CVD). All diagnoses were classified using the internationally accepted ICD definitions. In addition to documented diagnoses, the prescription of antihypertensive, lipid-lowering and anti-diabetic drugs was used to denote diagnosis of the relevant comorbidities.

> **Comments**
> - Assessment of the exposures of interest involved a National Patient Register. Although this negates the risk of recall bias, the use of data from a National Register carries its own issues and data is reliant on accurate coding and data input.

Statistical adjustment

Following data collection, statistical adjustments were made for sociodemographic variables including marital status, region of birth and educational level and for important comorbidities such as heart failure.

Results

A multivariable logistic regression model showed that type 2 diabetes, hypertension, hyperlipidaemia, obesity and chronic kidney disease were all associated with increased risk for severe Covid-19. The odds ratio and confidence intervals are illustrated in *Figure 2.4*. All associations remained significant after statistical adjustment for socioeconomic confounders (model 2). When adjusted for all diagnoses (model 3), the effect of hyperlipidaemia on the risk for severe Covid-19 lost statistical significance as the confidence interval crossed 1.

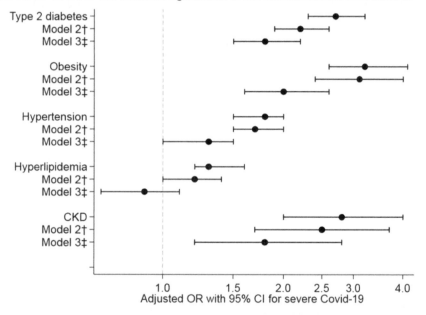

Figure 2.4. Adjusted OR with 95% CI for severe Covid-19 with type 2 diabetes, obesity, hypertension, hyperlipidaemia and CKD. Reproduced from *BMJ Open*, 11: e044486 under a CC BY 4.0 licence.

Conclusion

This study concluded that diabetes, obesity and hypertension were all independently associated with the risk for developing severe Covid-19.

2.9 Cohort studies

Cohort studies are longitudinal studies that follow participants over a period of time, often many years. During the study period, some of the participants will be exposed to risk factors and some will develop the health outcome of interest, usually a specific disease. Therefore, cohort studies allow us to characterise the association between exposures and health-related outcomes. They are of particular value in epidemiology and allow us to explore the effects of risk factors on disease development. As participants are recruited to the study before they develop the outcome of interest, these studies are prospective in nature. This is in contrast to case–control studies which are retrospective and take place after the disease has developed.

In order to perform a cohort study, a disease-free population is selected and the exposure is identified and defined. Examples of well-known exposures include smoking as a risk factor for lung cancer or hypertension as a risk for myocardial infarction. Following recruitment, participants are observed and the outcome is measured. Cohort studies provide superior evidence on disease causation than case–control studies. This is because in cohort studies, the exposure is known to have occurred prior to the outcome. Because of this, cohort studies are useful at identifying timelines between exposures and outcomes.

2.9.1 Relative risk

Cohort studies report results using the term **relative risk**. This is the probability of an outcome in the exposed group divided by the probability of an outcome in the unexposed group. The following worked example demonstrates the mathematical equation required to calculate relative risk and the interpretation of the value.

WORKED EXAMPLE
Hypoglycemia at admission is associated with inpatient mortality in Ugandan patients with severe sepsis

Ssekitoleko *et al.* (2011), *Crit Care Med*, **39**: 2271, doi.org/10.1097/CCM.0b013e3182227bd2

This study was a prospective cohort study investigating the association with hypoglycaemia and death in patients presenting to hospital with sepsis.

The results from the study are summarised in *Table 2.3*. In this example, the exposure of interest is hypoglycaemia and the outcome of interest is death.

Table 2.3: A 2×2 table outlining the frequency of death in those with and without hypoglycaemia in Ugandan inpatients with severe sepsis

	Died	Survived	Total
Hypoglycaemia	24	44	68
Euglycaemia	27	113	140

In order to calculate the relative risk (RR), the following steps are taken:

Risk for exposed = 24/68

Risk for unexposed = 27/140

RR = Risk for exposed / Risk for unexposed

RR = 0.35 / 0.19 = 1.8

Therefore, the risk of death in the hypoglycaemia group is 1.8 times greater than the risk of death in the euglycaemic group.

Comments

In general, the interpretation of the RR is as follows:

- RR >1: a higher proportion of people in the exposed group developed disease than those in the unexposed group. This suggests that the exposure is associated with increased risk for developing disease.

- RR = 1: there was an equal frequency of disease development in people exposed to the risk factor compared to people that were not exposed to the risk factor. This suggests that there is no association between the exposure and the development of the disease.

- RR <1: a lower proportion of people in the exposed group developed disease than those in the unexposed group. This suggests that the exposure is associated with decreased risk for developing disease.

In studies reporting negative outcomes such as mortality, the term 'hazard ratio' is sometimes used in place of relative risk. Both hazard ratio and relative risk are calculated using the same mathematical equation and both are interpreted in the same manner.

2.9.2 Disadvantages of cohort studies

Cohort studies are an effective way to investigate associations between exposures and outcomes. However, as is the case with all observational studies, there remains a risk for confounding. This risk is minimised by matching participants in the exposure and non-exposure groups. Other downsides to cohort studies are that they are costly and time-consuming. Therefore, they are not suitable for studying rare diseases or diseases that take a long time to develop. Attrition bias can present an issue in cohort studies, as some participants will drop out of the study and will become lost to follow-up. Other sources of bias may include change in participant behaviour due to involvement in a study and awareness of being observed; this is known as the Hawthorne effect.

WORKED EXAMPLE
Lung cancer and other causes of death in relation to smoking

Doll and Bradford Hill (1956), *BMJ*, **2**: 1071, doi.org/10.1136/bmj.2.5001.1071

Background

This is a landmark historical study that was the first to demonstrate a statistically strong association between smoking status and increased risk of death (from lung cancer and cardiovascular disease).

It was performed following the results of a case–control study showing that the risk of lung cancer was related to the number of cigarettes smoked per day. Following this report, the researchers designed a prospective cohort study to provide stronger evidence for this relationship.

Methodology

Questionnaires were sent to all of the doctors registered on the British Medical Register in 1951. In order to characterise the exposed and unexposed groups, participants identified themselves as current smokers, ex-smokers or never-smokers. In smokers and ex-smokers, data was collected surrounding the duration of smoking, the amount of tobacco smoked and the method of smoking.

In total, 59,600 men and women responded to the questionnaires. Participants under 35 and women were removed due to the low number of deaths and small sample size in these sub-populations, leaving 34,439 questionnaires for further analysis. Respondents were followed for a total of 50 years, with questionnaires sent out in 1957, 1966, 1971, 1978, 1991 and 2001.

In this study all the participants were UK doctors and the exposed group and unexposed group was identified by asking participants to report if they identified as: current smokers, ex-smokers, or never regularly smoked (defined as at least one cigarette a day for at least a year). Smokers and ex-smokers were asked when they started/stopped smoking, the amount of tobacco and method of smoking (pipes, cigarettes, etc).

> ### Comments
> - The large sample size and long follow-up period provides a strong body of evidence for the cause-and-effect relationship between smoking and lung cancer/cardiovascular disease. Furthermore, the collection of questionnaires at multiple time-points gives the opportunity to characterise the timing between smoking and disease development.

Results

The first results from this study were published in 1956. At this point, a total of 1714 deaths were reported in participants aged over 35. This included 81 people who died from lung cancer.

Ten years following study recruitment, 4597 deaths had been reported in the cohort. The results showed a strong association between the risk of death from lung cancer and the number of cigarettes smoked (3.15 per 1000 in men smoking 35 or more cigarettes a day compared to 0.07 per 1000 in non-smokers).

In the 50-year follow-up, the association between smoking and 12 types of cancer was made. Furthermore, information was published regarding years of life expectancy gained when smoking was stopped at different ages.

> ### Comments
> - The results from this ground-breaking cohort study were able to shed light upon the dangers of smoking, a concept that seems obvious for us today.

2.9.3 A comparison between cohort and case–control studies

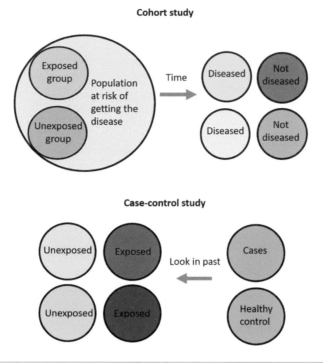

Figure 2.5. **A visual comparison of cohort versus case–control studies**. Circles represent groups of participants. In cohort studies an exposed group and unexposed group who are at risk of getting the disease are followed over time. In a case–control study cases are compared to healthy controls capable of catching the disease, and past exposure is assessed.

2.10 Randomised controlled trials

Randomised controlled trials (RCTs) are considered the gold standard of clinical studies to determine whether a treatment is safe and effective. They produce the highest quality of evidence on the cause and effect between an intervention and outcome, with the lowest impact of confounding variables. RCTs generally involve comparing participants receiving a novel treatment to a control group of participants who receive placebo or the current standard of care therapy. The different treatment conditions are known as '**arms**' of the trial. Most commonly, RCTs involve a 'treatment arm' vs. a 'control arm' but it is also possible to have many treatment arms, which could involve comparing two or more drugs to a control or varying the dose or treatment regime in different arms. Treatment regimens and outcome measures must be predefined so that we can assess if the researchers adhered to the protocol and so that results can be interpreted meaningfully.

2.10.1 Sample size estimation

Sample size estimation is an important concept in RCT study design and allows approximation of the number of subjects needed to be able to detect statistically significant changes between the two groups after an intervention. It is important to perform a sample size estimation for two main reasons. If the power calculation is not performed and the sample size is too big, the trial is inappropriately costly and time-consuming. If the sample size is too small, there is an increased risk of type I and II errors (discussed in *Section 3.9.2*).

2.10.2 Endpoints

The main aim of the trial is known as the primary endpoint and is decided on before the trial begins. It will be stated that 'the primary endpoint was met' if the trial meets the primary outcome with statistically significant results. For example, the primary endpoint may have been met if significantly more patients on drug A reached disease remission than those on placebo. In some RCTs, secondary endpoints are investigated. These are outcomes of interest but not the main aim. For example, in a trial investigating the effect of a new antihypertensive medication, the primary outcome may be a reduction in blood pressure. As hypertension is associated with cardiovascular disease, a relevant secondary endpoint may include the incidence of angina or myocardial infarction.

2.10.3 Blinding

Blinding refers to whether participants and/or researchers know which treatment arm subjects are allocated to. A trial is referred to as blinded if this information is kept from participants, double-blinded if this information is also masked from researchers, and triple-blinded if this includes data evaluators and statisticians. Where possible, blinding should be carried out to reduce the effects of bias. When trial participants are not blinded, knowledge of their treatment arm may affect their behaviour and response to treatment.

2.10.4 Randomisation

In a randomised trial, participants are randomly allocated to the different arms in the study, which means that they have an equal chance of ending up in each arm. This gives us statistical control over confounding variables that may influence the outcome; i.e. if the trial has a sufficient number of participants, the differences in characteristics between participants will be evenly distributed between the groups. Therefore, the population and selection bias will be minimised.

The method of randomisation is important to reduce bias; for instance, using date of birth or hospital number for assignment introduces bias, whereas a simple random number generator is a more appropriate method. Furthermore, with a smaller number of participants, simple randomisation may generate groups with a different characteristic in each case, therefore using block randomisation or stratification could be more suitable. The former ensures that the number of patients in each arm is balanced and the latter ensures the groups are similar in terms of certain characteristics such as age and sex.

Furthermore, allocation should be masked from the participants and researchers until the patient is already consented and ready to receive treatment. This is known as allocation concealment and is important to prevent bias as it could affect enrolment decisions.

2.10.5 **Control arm**

This can take many forms. If there is no standard-of-care treatment for the disease, the control may be a placebo. This means receiving no treatment or a sham treatment, which is something that appears the same as the treatment but has no pharmacological effect. An example of a sham treatment could be injecting saline into the knee joint to compare against a drug injection for treating rheumatoid arthritis.

If there is a standard-of-care treatment this may be used as the control and tested against the novel treatment of interest in the trial. This is preferred over the placebo control since depriving patients of treatment on a trial is not ethical (see discussion on ethics in *Section 4.6*).

2.10.6 **Superiority and non-inferiority trials**

The aim of the trial could be to show the treatment of interest is better than the standard-of-care which it is being compared to; this is known as a superiority trial. This contrasts to a non-inferiority trial where the aim is to see if the treatment is not unacceptably worse than the standard-of-care comparison. Therefore, non-inferiority studies do not demonstrate that a new treatment is more efficacious than the standard-of-care therapy. They are particularly useful when a new treatment offers benefits compared to the current standard-of-care therapy. For example, the new treatment may be cheaper, require less monitoring or be less invasive. In these cases, the new treatment does not need to be proven more efficacious than the standard-of-care therapy to become the preferred treatment option.

The distinction between planning a superiority and non-inferiority trial is necessary before trial commencement and there are different considerations for each type, such as sample size and analysis methods. Switching between superiority and non-inferiority analysis methods is generally not performed after the study has started but is nevertheless feasible in some cases.

2.10.7 **Intention to treat design**

Intention to treat is an important concept in RCT design. It is an analysis strategy that includes data from all randomised participants regardless of whether they deviated or withdrew from the study. There are two main purposes of an intention to treat analysis.

The intention to treat approach assumes that the different arms are similar apart from random variation. Therefore, if data analysis is not performed on the groups produced by the randomisation process, the two groups are no longer similar and an element of bias is introduced. For example, in a study comparing the efficacy of surgery and chemotherapy in patients with cancer, it might be tempting to exclude participants in the surgical arm who died pre-operatively. If these subjects were excluded, the participants allocated to receive surgery may have a falsely low mortality rate and surgery may incorrectly appear to be more effective than chemotherapy.

The second purpose of intention to treat analyses is that they allow for protocol deviation and non-compliance. This is important because most types of protocol deviation occur in routine clinical practice and therefore should not be ignored. For example, data from participants who are not fully adherent with the allocated medication should be included in the overall analysis. This is very important because in real life, patients commonly miss doses of prescribed medications. Therefore, if medication non-adherence was ignored, the effects of the medication will be overestimated when prescribed in the general population.

2.10.8 Disadvantages of RCTs

The main drawbacks of RCTs are their economical and labour burden. Furthermore, results may not be generalisable to the whole patient population due to volunteer bias and strict inclusion/exclusion criteria. This means that subjects who enrol onto trials may be more compliant with medication and have fewer comorbidities, which may not be representative of the population as a whole. Due to the long trial run time, results from RCTs may lose relevance due to changes in practice by the time of publication.

WORKED EXAMPLE
Apixaban versus warfarin in patients with atrial fibrillation

Granger *et al.* (2011), *NEJM*, doi.org/10.1056/NEJMoa1107039

Background
Patients with atrial fibrillation (AF) are at increased risk of ischaemic stroke. Warfarin is a well-established treatment for AF and has been shown to reduce the risk of stroke by two-thirds. Directly acting oral anticoagulants (DOACs), including apixaban, carry advantages over warfarin such as reduced monitoring requirements and fewer drug and food interactions.

In the Apixaban for Reduction in Stroke and Other Thromboembolic Events in Atrial Fibrillation (ARISTOTLE) trial, investigators compared warfarin and apixaban in preventing stroke and systemic embolism in patients with AF.

Methods
This trial was a double-blind, randomised control trial. Enrolled participants were randomised to receive apixaban or warfarin.

The primary objective was to determine whether apixaban was non-inferior to warfarin in the prevention of stroke and systemic embolism.

The primary safety outcome was to compare the rates of major bleeding in participants on warfarin versus apixaban. Major bleeding was defined using well-established criteria published by the International Society on Thrombosis and Haemostasis (ISTH). The key secondary outcome was death from any cause.

Both primary and secondary outcomes were analysed using an intention to treat approach.

> **Comments**
> - The primary endpoint was a non-inferiority outcome. In this case, apixaban offers benefits over warfarin such as reduced food and medication interactions and reduced need for blood monitoring. Therefore, a non-inferiority design was appropriate as apixaban could be the preferred treatment provided that it is no less efficacious than warfarin.
> - Outcomes were clearly defined.
> - The study used an intention to treat analysis approach.

Eligible patients had AF or atrial flutter at enrolment or two previous episodes recorded using electrocardiography. For enrolment into the study, participants had to have at least one other risk factor for the development of stroke. These factors were clearly defined by the study team.

Exclusion criteria were clearly stated and included mitral stenosis, concurrent dual antiplatelet use and severe renal insufficiency.

A stratified randomisation technique was used to allocate participants to the different arms according to previous warfarin use and clinical site.

> **Comments**
> - Inclusion and exclusion criteria need to be met before subject enrolment into RCTs. This is important in all RCTs and ensures that the appropriate group of participants are enrolled into the RCT.
> - There are different techniques to randomise participants into each arm of an RCT. Stratified randomisation groups patients into strata according to clinical features that may influence outcome risk (e.g. previous use of warfarin in this study). Within each stratum, participants are allocated to treatment arms using a different randomisation technique. Stratified randomisation aims to prevent the imbalance of known confounding factors between groups.

The primary non-inferiority outcome required that treatment with apixaban was associated with at least 50% of the relative risk reduction in the incidence of stroke compared to those on warfarin.

A sample size calculation was performed prior to study commencement and estimated that 18,000 participants would need to be recruited to reach the study endpoint.

> **Comments**
> - The sample size estimation required data from previous RCTs in warfarin. In this case, data from six major RCTs was included. More information about sample size estimation is outlined in *Chapter 3*.
> - Different calculations are needed to estimate sample size in non-inferiority versus superiority RCTs.

Results
In total, 18,201 participants were recruited at 1034 clinical sites across 39 countries. Participants allocated to both arms were similar with respect to age, gender, comorbidities and concurrent medications.

> **Comments**
> - This is a large sample size which includes participants from different geographical locations.
> - The groups are well matched with regard to demographic characteristics and comorbidities. This is important because many of these factors have the potential to act as confounding factors (by influencing both exposure and outcome).

The primary outcome of stroke or systemic embolism occurred in 212 participants in the apixaban group (1.27% per year) and 265 participants in the warfarin group (1.60% per year). The hazard ratio in the apixaban group was 0.79; 95% CI 0.66, P <0.001. Primary outcome data is summarised in *Table 2.4*.

Table 2.4: A summary of primary outcome data including the incidence of stroke and systemic embolism

Primary outcome	Apixaban group (n = 9120)		Warfarin group (n = 9081)		Hazard ratio (HR) (95% CI)	P value
	Patients with event (no.)	Event rate (%/yr)	Patients with event (no.)	Event rate (%/yr)		
Stroke	199	1.19	250	1.51	0.79 (0.65–0.95)	0.01
Ischaemic or uncertain stroke	162	0.97	175	1.05	0.92 (0.74–1.13)	0.42
Haemorrhagic stroke	40	0.24	78	0.47	0.51 (0.35–0.75)	<0.001
Systemic embolism	15	0.09	17	0.10	0.87 (0.44–1.75)	0.70
Total	**212**	**1.27**	**265**	**1.60**	**0.79 (0.66–0.95)**	**0.01**

All-cause mortality and major bleeding rates were lower in the apixaban arm than the warfarin arm (HR 0.89; 95% CI 0.80–0.99, HR 0.69; 95% CI 0.60–0.80). Both of these outcomes reached statistical significance (P <0.05).

The reduction in primary outcomes with apixaban was consistent across all of the major predefined subgroups, which included ethnicity, BMI and the presence of heart failure. In total, 21 subgroups were considered.

> **Comments**
> - In this study, participants on apixaban were 0.79 times as likely to reach the primary outcome (stroke or systemic embolism) than participants on warfarin. Although the primary outcome was non-inferiority, the study also concluded that apixaban was superior to warfarin in preventing stroke and systemic embolism.
> - Apixaban was associated with significantly reduced mortality and major bleeding compared to warfarin.
> - The consistency of results across the major subgroups suggests that the study conclusions are generalisable across different populations.

Conclusion

In participants with AF, apixaban was associated with reduced risk for stroke, bleeding and mortality compared to warfarin.

Compared to warfarin, the relative reduction in the risk for stroke or systemic embolism was 21%, major bleeding 31% and death 11%. As compared to warfarin, for every 1000 patients treated with apixaban for a total of 1.8 years, a stroke was prevented in 6 individuals, major bleeding in 15 and death in 8.

> Comments
> - Overall, this study was a landmark RCT providing evidence for the efficacy and safety of apixaban when compared to warfarin.

2.11 Systematic reviews

Systematic reviews attempt to identify all existing research studies which answer a specific research question. The purpose of the systematic review is to provide a summary of all of the available research and to provide the most reliable source of evidence to guide clinical practice.

Studies are selected on a systematic search of the literature databases with pre-specified eligibility criteria. Typical eligibility criteria include keywords used to search publications, e.g. drug name, type of study and whether it was a controlled study. These differ from narrative reviews which have not been rigorously screened based on predefined search criteria, which include studies selected by the author and have the downside of selection bias based on author opinions.

2.11.1 Useful databases

Databases are used to store the results from systematic reviews. The Cochrane Library is the most well-known database and contains over 7500 systematic reviews. Cochrane is a not-for-profit organisation whose goal is to provide high-quality evidence for healthcare choices.

Other useful databases include PROSPERO, Medline and Embase. These databases accept registrations for new studies including systematic reviews, rapid reviews and umbrella reviews. This allows researchers to enter information about their own new work, confirm it is novel and therefore ensure that they are not replicating previously published work.

2.11.2 Performing a systematic review

Below is a step-by-step guide to performing a systematic review. The whole process involves extensive work and usually takes between 6 months and a year.

1. **Define a research question**

The first step in a systematic review is to define a research question. It is important to keep this brief and specific.

There are two common models used to construct a research question:

- PICO (Population, Intervention, Comparison and Outcomes)

The PICO format is the most commonly used format in evidence-based clinical practice.

Example: What is the risk of infection for targeted synthetic disease-modifying agents compared to biological therapies for treating rheumatoid arthritis?

P: patients with rheumatoid arthritis

I: targeted synthetic disease-modifying agents

C: biological therapies

O: risk of infection

- SPIDER (Sample, Phenomenon of Interest, Design, Evaluation, Research type)

SPIDER is generally preferred for qualitative and mixed methods research (qualitative research is discussed in more detail in *Chapter 6*).

Example: What are arthritis patients' experiences of attending outpatient appointments?

S: patients with rheumatoid arthritis

P of **I:** outpatient appointments

D: questionnaire, focus group, observational study

E: experience

R: qualitative

Prior to moving to step two, do a preliminary search to validate the proposed question and avoid duplication of previously addressed questions.

2. **Develop a protocol**

A protocol must be developed prior to data collection. A good protocol outlines the methodology involved in the study and defines the three following features:

- Research question
- Inclusion and exclusion criteria

It is important to clearly define the eligibility criteria prior to data collection. This avoids bias during the search. Important inclusion and exclusion criteria to consider include study population, comparison groups and outcome of interest. Inclusion criteria must also state study date and design. For example, it might be decided that all clinical trials in the area will be included in the analysis. If higher-quality data exists, only RCTs might be selected.

- Methodology

  The protocol must clearly define the search strategy, search terms, method for quality assessment and study selection. Methods for data extraction, analysis and the synthesis of results must be clearly stated.

  It is very important to clearly define the search terms in the protocol. When planning a search, there is a delicate balance between specificity (retrieving relevant papers) and sensitivity (attempting to retrieve all research on the question). When the search criteria are too broad, an unmanageable number of papers may be returned. When the search criteria are narrow, there is a risk of missing important studies.

3. **Start searching**

   Use databases to perform electronic literature searches. Example databases include PubMed, Medline, Cochrane Library, Embase, Web of Science and Google Scholar. Only databases relevant to your topic should be searched.

   It is important to log searches and the number of papers retrieved from each search. Search using AND to bring up papers including both search terms and OR for synonyms. However, some databases do not use Boolean logic so alter search strategy based on the database.

   It is important to delete duplicate studies when searches retrieve the same paper. This can be done by collecting all records into a citation manager such as Endnote and then exporting into an Excel sheet as a second check.

   In addition to database searches, manual searching can be performed to ensure that all relevant papers have been retrieved. This may involve asking scientists working in the field or searching reference lists, library resources and conference proceedings.

4. **Screen and select studies**

   After returning a study, scan the title and abstract to decide if it is relevant. Irrelevant studies should be logged and excluded. After the initial screen, the full text should be read to determine whether it fulfils the predefined eligibility criteria. More than one person should independently select studies. When there is disagreement between the reviewers, a predefined method should be used to create consensus.

   When selecting studies, the validity should be assessed. Important factors to consider include the method of randomisation and blinding. Sources of bias should be considered. Studies that do not meet the criteria for adequate validity are excluded and reasons why should be stated.

   When selecting studies to include in a systematic review, standardised assessment tools such as the Joanna Briggs Institute Appraisal Tools checklist (https://jbi. global/critical-appraisal-tools) can provide a structured approach.

5. **Extract data**

   Data should be extracted exactly as it appears; this can be done with a data extraction form or systematic review software. Two or more independent reviewers should be responsible for this step.

6. **Analyse results**

   This is the difficult part! Summarise the differences between the studies and interpret the findings, considering the validity assessment. This can be achieved by assessing the rigour of the results from different studies. Important considerations include sample size, randomisation method and blinding method.

   Contradictory studies present the biggest challenge when interpreting results. Methods to reconcile contradictory findings should be defined in the protocol.

   When outcome data is consistent and study data is accessible, a meta-analysis may be performed. This is a specific subtype of systematic review that employs statistical methods to analyse results. When a meta-analysis is possible, it provides a powerful method of estimating the effect size of an intervention and increases the generalisability of the results from different studies.

7. **Write up results and disseminate findings**

   Summarise your findings and highlight any inconsistencies and important future research to be done.

   Authors should report methodology accurately – one way to do this is by using a PRISMA flow diagram which describes each step in detail. A PRISMA diagram is shown in *Figure 2.5* in the next worked example.

2.11.3 **Meta-analysis**

Meta-analyses are a subset of systematic review that assess the overall effect size of an intervention. In contrast to traditional studies that tell you whether an intervention has a statistically significant effect, meta-analyses can tell you the direction and magnitude of the treatment effect by pooling results from multiple studies. For example, a meta-analysis of studies investigating the use of an antihypertensive can estimate the average reduction in blood pressure with treatment.

Meta-analyses are useful to reconcile studies with conflicting results. They are statistically strong as they include a large and diverse cohort. By pooling smaller studies, they offer the possibility of increasing statistical power to detect small treatment effects.

To perform a meta-analysis, search processes and study selection follow the same steps as summarised above. In contrast to systematic reviews, all studies included in a meta-analysis must be similar in type. This is important in order to combine results.

Most commonly, RCTs are used for meta-analysis as they produce the highest quality of evidence. The most common measures for effect size are relative risk (RR) and odds ratio (OR) for dichotomous data and standardised mean difference (SMD) for continuous data (see https://training.cochrane.org/handbook for further information).

In order to combine the results from different studies included in the meta-analysis, the effect size should be weighted based on the strength of the evidence. Statistically, this is usually denoted by the inverse of the studies variance. Broadly speaking, studies with larger sample sizes have a lower variance and therefore carry higher weights. When performing meta-analysis, larger studies with more participants generally carry higher weighting than smaller studies. It is important to note that other factors affect the variance and more information on this is summarised in *Chapter 3*.

There are two models which can be used when combining study results in a meta-analysis: a fixed effects model and a random effects model.

The **fixed effects model** assumes that there is one true effect size and that this is the same in all studies. Therefore, the model assumes that there are no differences in study population, selection criteria and treatment method between all studies that are included in the meta-analysis. As all studies are assumed to be estimating the same effect size, weights are assigned purely on the basis of sample size. Therefore, large studies are given more weight than smaller studies.

The **random effects model** assumes that there are true differences between study results due to differences in population selection, methods and treatment protocols between studies. For example, the effect size of a treatment might be higher in one study because the selected population is older, multimorbid or because the study treatment regime is slightly longer or more intensive. The random effects model attempts to take these differences into account and aims to estimate the mean value and the distribution of true effects. This is summarised by the heterogeneity parameter which quantifies the distribution of true effects around the mean overall effect. Multiple statistical methods can be used to calculate the heterogeneity parameter including the I^2 statistic. This is discussed in *Section 3.11.3*.

2.11.4 Forest plot

Results from a meta-analysis are usually displayed in a **forest plot**. This illustrates the weighted effect size and confidence interval for each individual study and the pooled effect size and confidence interval for combined data. Statistical programs are available to calculate effect sizes, such as the Review Manager (RevMan) program. The worked example below takes us through the interpretation of a forest plot.

2.11.5 Limitations of meta-analysis

Although meta-analyses are useful tools to summarise the results from multiple RCTs, there are limitations that should be considered in their interpretation. Firstly, there are often significant differences between the design and conduct of RCTs included in meta-analysis. For example, there may be differences in study population, treatment protocols and outcomes of interest. In some cases, the studies are sufficiently different that combining their results would not be valid. Differences in study design may result in dissimilarity between the results of different studies. This is known as heterogeneity. Assessing the degree of between-studies heterogeneity is an important step in meta-analysis. This can be performed using statistical methods (discussed in *Section 3.11.3*). The validity of meta-analysis is dependent on the RCTs. When low-quality studies are included in the analysis, the result will be of poor quality. This can be limited by defining strict inclusion criteria and including high-quality studies. An important issue in meta-analysis design and interpretation is **publication bias**. This refers to the fact that studies reporting positive results are more likely to be published than those reporting negative results. The presence of publication bias may overestimate the magnitude and effect size of the meta-analysis results. This is discussed in more detail in the worked example and in *Section 3.11.2*.

WORKED EXAMPLE
Angiotensin-converting enzyme inhibitors reduce mortality in hypertension: a meta-analysis of randomized clinical trials of renin–angiotensin–aldosterone system inhibitors involving 158,998 patients

van Vark *et al.* (2012), *Eur Heart J*, 33: 2088, doi.org/10.1093/eurheartj/ehs075

Background
Renin–angiotensin–aldosterone system (RAAS) inhibitors are common antihypertensives that are well established to reduce cardiovascular mortality in patients with hypertension. This meta-analysis set out to investigate the effect of RAAS inhibitors, including angiotensin-converting enzyme inhibitors (ACEi) and AT1 receptor blockers (ARB), on all-cause mortality in patients with hypertension.

Search method and study selection
The meta-analysis aimed to include all publicly available morbidity–mortality prospective RCTs that compared treatment with an ACEi or ARB with control treatment. In order to do this, they performed a systematic search of OVID MEDLINE and ISI Web of Science, using key words including "anti-hypertensive agents", "angiotensin receptor blockers", "angiotensin-converting enzyme inhibitors" and "hypertension". Studies published between January 2000 and March 2011 were included. Each trial was independently evaluated by two investigators to assess for patient population, study treatment and endpoints.

Endpoint definition
The study clearly defined the endpoint as all-cause mortality and cardiovascular mortality during long-term follow-up. The authors measured this using mortality incident rate (IR). This allowed comparison between different studies with different follow-up periods.

Comments
- The authors clearly defined their search strategy including the terms used and the databases searched. This is summarised in the PRISMA flow diagram (*Figure 2.5*) which also gives an overview of study selection in the meta-analysis. As illustrated, studies were first screened for relevance. Following this, a more detailed review was performed and studies were selected if they met eligibility criteria. The number of studies retrieved and excluded at each step is summarised in the diagram.
- In all systematic reviews and meta-analyses, it is important for at least two independent researchers to evaluate studies meeting the eligibility criteria.

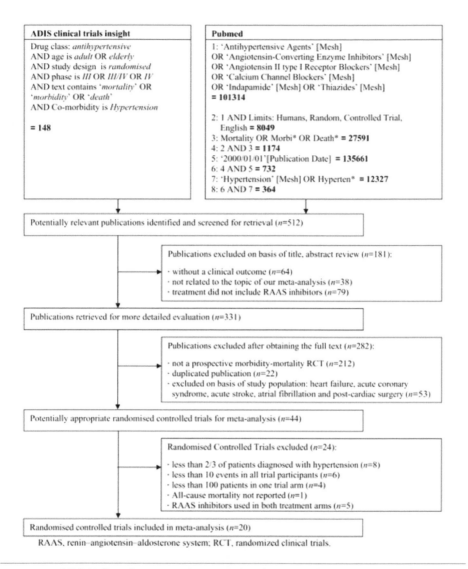

Figure 2.6. PRISMA flow diagram outlining study selection in the meta-analysis.
Reproduced from *Eur Heart J*, 33: 2088 with permission from Oxford University Press.

Results

During a mean follow-up period of 4.3 years, 6284 patients assigned to a RAAS inhibitor group reached the endpoint of all-cause mortality compared to 8777 in the control group. This corresponded to mortality incidence rates of 20.9 and 23.3 deaths per 1000 patient years, respectively. When the results from the 20 trials were pooled, there was a statistically significant 5% reduction in all-cause mortality (HR 0.95; 95% CI 0.91–1.00, $P = 0.032$). The degree of heterogeneity in the treatment effect was low between all included trials (I^2=15%).

There was no funnel-plot asymmetry demonstrated; this indicates a lower chance of publication bias.

Comments

- In this meta-analysis, the hazard ratio was 0.95 for all-cause mortality in subjects on RAAS inhibitors. This means that participants prescribed a RAAS inhibitor had a 5% lower risk of death than those in the control group. This is statistically significant, as the *P* value is less than 0.05.

- Meta-analyses usually report the degree of heterogeneity between the results from different studies. There are different measurements that can be used to characterise heterogeneity. In this case, the I² statistic was used. This is a statistic that estimates the degree of the between-study variance that is explained by heterogeneity rather than chance. The higher the I² statistic, the larger the between-study heterogeneity. In this case, the heterogeneity parameter is low. This indicates that the true effect differences between individual studies are similar. Heterogeneity is discussed in more detail in *Section 3.11.3.*

- Publication bias is an important issue in the interpretation of meta-analyses. Publications with positive results are more likely to be published than those with negative results. By omitting the results from negative studies, there is a risk of false positive meta-analysis results. A **funnel plot** is used to characterise the degree of publication bias. It is a scatter plot of the effect sizes from individual studies against a measure of the studies' precision or size. In a funnel plot, the smaller studies are plotted at the bottom of the graph and the larger studies are at the top. In the absence of publication bias and between-study heterogeneity, the scatter plot will appear as a symmetrical inverted funnel. When there is bias (including publication bias) or significant heterogeneity, the funnel plot will become asymmetrical. In this case, the funnel plot was symmetrical, indicating a low chance of bias. Publication bias is discussed in more detail in *Section 3.11.2.*

The study results are illustrated in *Figure 2.7.*

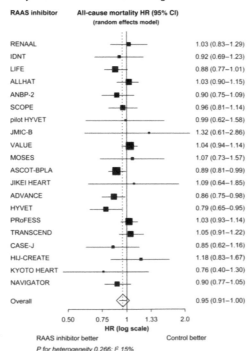

Figure 2.7. Forest plot summarising the hazard ratio for all-cause mortality across all studies included in the meta-analysis. Reproduced from *Eur Heart J*, 33: 2088 with permission from Oxford University Press.

Comments

- Results from meta-analyses are usually illustrated in a forest plot. The horizontal axis represents the statistic of interest; in this case, the log of the hazard ratio for all-cause mortality. Conventionally, a vertical line is drawn to illustrate the line of null effect. This is the line where there is no association between the intervention and outcome of interest.

- The results from each study are depicted by individual horizontal lines. In this worked example, 20 individual studies are included in the forest plot. The results from each study include a point effect estimate which is represented by a black box. The size of the box gives a representation of the weighting of each study, usually determined by study size. The larger the black box, the larger the study and the higher the weighting to the overall result. The horizontal line intersecting each box represents the boundaries of the 95% confidence intervals from each study. The longer the line, the less precise the estimate of the effect. When the horizontal line crosses the "line of null effect" (in this case, a log HR of 1) this indicates that the study has not produced a statistically significant result.

- The pooled result from the meta-analysis is represented by the diamond at the bottom of the plot. This is the most important component of the forest plot and represents the point estimate and confidence intervals from the pooled analysis. If the diamond crosses the line of null effect, there is no statistically significant effect of intervention. In this example, the diamond touches but does not cross the line of null effect. Therefore, the result is considered significant.

Conclusion

In conclusion, this study demonstrated a significant 5% reduction in all-cause mortality in participants prescribed RAAS inhibitors for hypertension. The study went on to show that the reduction in mortality was explained entirely from ACEi which were associated with a 10% reduction in mortality, compared to ARBs which were associated with a 0% mortality reduction.

Comments

- This study showed that ACEi were associated with a reduction in all-cause mortality in hypertensive patients.

2.12 Summary of study types

Throughout this chapter we have discussed the different types of study design, including their strengths and weaknesses. The studies described are summarised in the table below.

Table 2.5: A summary of study designs including a description of the study type and study advantages and disadvantages

Study type	Description	Advantages	Disadvantages
Meta-analysis	Subtype of systematic review that uses statistical methods to pool the results from multiple clinical studies	Large degree of statistical power due to pooling of results from different studies Allows estimation of magnitude and effect size of intervention	Limited by quality of existing RCTs Results prone to publication bias Validity and generalisability due to heterogeneity between studies
Systematic review	Descriptive analysis of all available studies that answer a specific research question	Can be used when a meta-analysis is not possible, i.e. when there is a significant degree of study heterogeneity	Unable to quantify the effect of an intervention
Randomised controlled trial	Experimental study usually comparing the efficacy of a new therapy to standard-of-care therapy or placebo	Provides the highest amount of evidence with the lowest impact of confounding variables	Expensive, resource-intensive and lengthy Not suitable for some scenarios which would be unethical Strict eligibility criteria may result in a sample that is not representative of the population Susceptible to certain types of bias, including attrition bias and volunteer bias
Cohort study	Observational study characterising the relationship between exposure and the development of an outcome, usually a disease	Provides the highest level of evidence for the association between exposure and outcome in observational studies Good for rare exposures	Study population selection can lead to bias Not suitable for rare diseases or diseases that take a long time to develop More expensive than case–control studies Subjects may be lost to follow-up
Case–control study	Observational study characterising past exposures in people who have already developed an outcome, usually a disease, compared to those who haven't	Cheaper than cohort studies Good for the study of rare diseases	Data is collected retrospectively and therefore prone to recall bias Impossible to determine temporal relationship between exposure and outcome

Cross-sectional study	Estimation of prevalence of exposure and outcome in a sample	Cheap, easy and fast to conduct	Snapshot may not be representative
		Multiple exposures and outcomes may be measured	Impossible to measure incidence
			Cannot establish causality or temporal association between exposure and outcome
		Prevalence data can be useful in planning public health interventions	Prone to bias including non-response and recall bias
Case report	Describes unusual or novel clinical cases	May be first description of a novel disease or outcome	Results are not generalisable due to the effects of bias and chance
		Can highlight important learning points	

2.13 Further reading and other resources

Cochrane database: www.cochrane.org

Health Data Research UK: www.hdruk.ac.uk

National Institute for Health and Care Research: www.nihr.ac.uk

PROSPERO: www.crd.york.ac.uk/prospero

Research Design Service London: www.rds-london.nihr.ac.uk

UK Biobank: www.ukbiobank.ac.uk

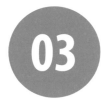

CHAPTER 3

Statistics

Introduction

Statistics is the science of collecting, analysing, interpreting and presenting data. This chapter will provide a concise overview of some of the key concepts involved in statistics along with worked examples highlighting the application of different statistical methods.

3.2 **Obtaining and describing data**

3.2.1 Types of data

Different types of statistical methods are used to analyse different types of data. The main types of data are summarised below.

Numerical data

This is quantitative data. The two main types include continuous and discrete data.

- **Continuous data**
  - Continuous data can take any numerical value and can be meaningfully subdivided into finer levels. Continuous data is usually measured on a scale or a continuum.
  - Measurements such as height and weight fall into this category, e.g. 1.54m and 53.4kg.
- **Discrete data**
  - Discrete data can only take certain numerical values, usually integers. The discrete values cannot be subdivided and therefore only a limited number of values is possible.
  - Examples include number of people or number of hospital visits. In these examples, it is not possible to subdivide integers into smaller increments such as half a person or half a hospital visit.

Categorical data

This is data that has been grouped into categories on the basis of qualitative features. The types include nominal, ordinal and binary data.

- **Nominal data**
  - Nominal data is grouped into categories that cannot be ordered.
  - Examples include blood group or ethnicity.
- **Ordinal data**
  - Ordinal data is grouped into categories that can be ordered.
  - Examples include tumour stage.
- **Binary/dichotomous data**
  - Binary data refers to data where there are only two possible values (e.g. 0 or 1) or two possible categories (e.g. dead or alive).

3.2.2 Obtaining data, i.e. sampling

Clinical researchers are usually interested in populations. Populations are defined as groups of individuals who share a common characteristic or condition, usually a disease. For example, a researcher investigating rheumatoid arthritis is interested in all patients who have been diagnosed with this condition. In clinical research, it is generally not feasible to study an entire population, and therefore a subset or sample of the population is recruited to the study. The study reports the results obtained from the

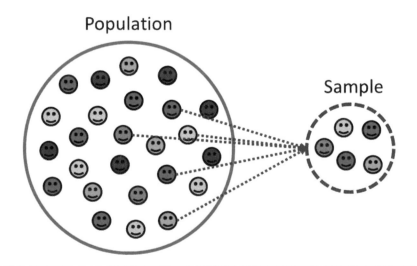

Figure 3.1. Obtaining a sample from a population. A sample is a subset of the population that is included in a research study. The sample should be representative of the population in order for researchers to infer conclusions regarding the wider population.

sample (the sample estimate) and this is used to estimate the value in the population (the population parameter). In order for the sample estimate to accurately reflect the population parameter, the individuals in the sample must be representative of the individuals in the population (see the sampling section below for more details on how this is achieved). When the sample is not representative of the general population, the sample estimate does not equal the population parameter. This is sampling error. When significant sampling error occurs, the results of the study cannot be generalised to the overall population, thus limiting the external validity of the study.

Sampling methods

Different methods are used to select a sample for inclusion into a clinical study. Three examples of sampling method are summarised below.

- **Simple random sampling:** in this scenario, every member of the population has an equal probability of selection into the sample. Theoretically, a researcher may have a list of all of the patients diagnosed with Goodpasture's syndrome. In this case, the list is called the "sampling frame". In order to select a sample, individuals are randomly drawn from the list using methods such as a random number generator. In reality, the entire population of patients with a defined disease, such as Goodpasture's syndrome, is not usually available for possible recruitment and this type of sampling is generally not feasible.

- **Stratified random sampling:** this is a modification of random sampling. In this scenario, the whole population is divided into homogenous strata according to demographic or clinical factors (examples include gender, ethnicity and comorbidity). After the population are divided into strata, the researcher selects a random sample of individuals from each stratum to be included into the clinical trial.

  Stratified random sampling is a widely-used sampling method in clinical trials. It allows researchers to study effect sizes between different groups and allows sampling from under-represented categories.

- **Convenience sampling:** in this method, participants are recruited on the basis of availability and ease of access. For example, in a study investigating patients with rheumatoid arthritis, individuals attending outpatient rheumatology clinics within the study period are recruited. Convenience sampling is a widely used method for subject recruitment as it is easy, cheap and quick. On the downside, convenience sampling may introduce an element of bias into subject recruitment. For example, individuals attending clinic may be more compliant with medical treatments than the individuals who do not attend their appointments.

Accuracy versus precision

When obtaining a sample estimate, it is important to consider its accuracy and its precision.

Precision: a measure of how close measured values are to each other
Accuracy: a measure of how close the sample estimate is expected to be to the population parameter

3.2.3 Measures of central location

Measures of central location represent the average values in a dataset. The most commonly used measures include the mean, median and mode.

The **arithmetic mean** is the best-known average value. It is calculated by summing all of the values in a dataset and dividing by the total number of values. The mean is easy to calculate and convenient to use in many contexts. By considering all values in a dataset, the mean is the most sensitive method to measure an average. The main disadvantage to using the mean is that it is highly influenced by extreme values (or outliers).

The **median** lies at the midpoint of all values in a dataset when they are ordered numerically. Therefore, 50% of values in a dataset are greater than the median value and 50% of values are lower. The median is not influenced by extreme values and is preferable to the mean when outliers are present.

The **mode** is the value that occurs most frequently in a dataset. The mode is not commonly used as a measure of average as it is not generally representative of the data. It is, however, useful to know whether a dataset has one or two modal values. When a dataset has one modal value, it is described as unimodal.

3.2.4 Measures of spread

Common measures of spread include the range, interquartile range, variance and standard deviation.

The **range** is the difference between the largest and smallest value in a dataset. It is very simple to calculate but may not be representative of the dataset, particularly when outliers are present.

The **interquartile range (IQR)** is calculated by ordering the dataset, dividing it into quartiles and calculating the difference between the bottom and top quartile. The IQR therefore indicates where the middle 50% of the data lie. The IQR is not influenced by outliers and therefore is a useful measure of spread when data is not symmetrically distributed.

A **box and whisker plot** is a common method to display the median, IQR and the range of a dataset. Its interpretation is outlined in *Figure 3.2*.

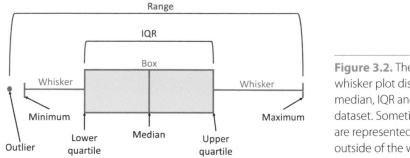

Figure 3.2. The box and whisker plot displays the median, IQR and range of a dataset. Sometimes, outliers are represented as points outside of the whiskers.

The symmetry of the box and whisker plot gives useful information regarding the distribution of the data. This is discussed in more detail in *Section 3.3.1*.

The **variance** measures the degree to which individual values in a dataset deviate from the mean. The larger the variance, the larger the spread of the data.

The variance is calculated using the following steps:

1. Subtract the mean from each value in the dataset

2. Square each of the differences and add all of the squares together

3. Divide the sum of the squares by the number of values in the dataset minus 1

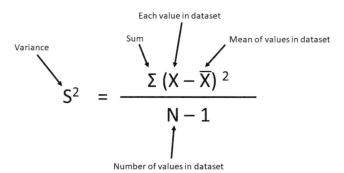

$$S^2 = \frac{\Sigma (X - \overline{X})^2}{N - 1}$$

Figure 3.3. Equation to calculate the variance of values in a dataset.

The **standard deviation (SD)** is derived from the variance and is a very commonly reported measure of spread. It is calculated by performing the square root of the variance. Therefore, the larger the standard deviation, the larger the spread of the data. Both the variance and the SD are calculated using computer programs, such as SPSS or GraphPad.

WORKED EXAMPLE
Sphingosine-1-phosphate and CRP as potential combination biomarkers in discrimination of COPD with community-acquired pneumonia and acute exacerbation of COPD

Hsu *et al.* (2022) *Resp Res, 23*: 63, doi.org/10.1186/s12931-022-01991-1

Study aim

This study evaluated the use of the blood marker sphingosine-1-phosphate (S1P) to differentiate between community-acquired pneumonia and acute exacerbation in patients with COPD.

Results

The following box and whisker plots show the S1P readings in COPD patients with acute exacerbation (AE) compared to those with pneumonia (Pn).

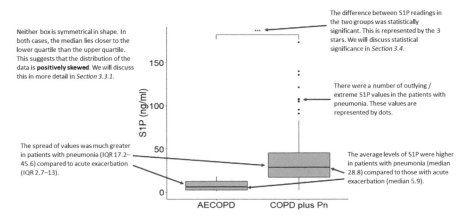

Neither box is symmetrical in shape. In both cases, the median lies closer to the lower quartile than the upper quartile. This suggests that the distribution of the data is **positively skewed**. We will discuss this in more detail in *Section 3.3.1*.

The difference between S1P readings in the two groups was statistically significant. This is represented by the 3 stars. We will discuss statistical significance in *Section 3.4*.

There were a number of outlying / extreme S1P values in the patients with pneumonia. These values are represented by dots.

The spread of values was much greater in patients with pneumonia (IQR 17.2–45.6) compared to acute exacerbation (IQR 2.7–13).

The average levels of S1P were higher in patients with pneumonia (median 28.8) compared to those with acute exacerbation (median 5.9).

Figure 3.4. A worked example of the interpretation of two box and whisker plots. Image reproduced under a CC BY 4.0 licence.

Comments

- This example nicely illustrates the importance of choosing the correct measure of average and spread to describe your study data. In this case, the median and IQR were used because the data was skewed and because there were a number of outlying data points. In this example, it would have been inappropriate to use the mean and SD, which are highly influenced by outlying values.

3.3 | Distribution, probability and confidence intervals

3.3.1 Types of distribution

Throughout this book, we will consider two main types of distribution:

1. **Probability distribution**: this is a mathematical distribution that gives us the predicted probability of an outcome occurring. Probability distributions have important applications in medical statistics, including in the calculation of confidence intervals and in hypothesis testing.

2. **Frequency distribution**: this gives us the observed frequency of a particular data point in a study or experiment. A frequency distribution is plotted on a histogram after data has been collected. In clinical research, quantitative data can follow a variety of different frequency distributions. These are important to consider because they influence hypothesis testing and statistical analysis (discussed in *Section 3.5*).

Probability and probability distributions

Probability is an important concept in statistics. It is defined as a measure of uncertainty, i.e. how likely something is to occur. Numerically, it is usually expressed as a value between 0 and 1, where 0 is impossible and 1 is certain.

Probability distributions are theoretical distributions that show the probability of all of the possible values of a random variable. For example, imagine the probability distribution when rolling two dice. Each die has a 1 in 6 (0.17) probability of rolling any number, one to six. When rolling two dice, the sum of the rolled values on the two dice will form the probability distribution illustrated below.

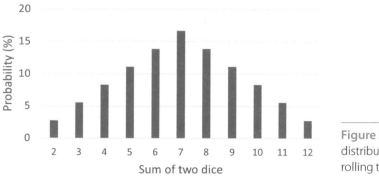

Figure 3.5. Probability distribution for sum of rolling two dice.

As you can see, seven is the most likely number to roll and occurs in 6 out of 36 rolls (17% of rolls). Conversely, rolling a two is much less likely and will only occur in 1 out of 36 rolls (3% of rolls). In this example, the probability distribution gives us the predicted outcome of rolling each number. If an experiment was performed where two dice were rolled 50 times and the results were plotted, the frequency distribution would differ from the probability distribution due to the effects of chance. As the number of rolls increases, the frequency distribution approaches the shape of the probability distribution.

The normal distribution

Probability and frequency distributions can follow a **normal distribution**. This is a symmetrical distribution that follows a bell-shaped curve with a single peak. Mathematically, the normal distribution follows a Gaussian curve and is symmetrical around the mean value. When data is normally distributed, the mean, median and mode are equal. The width of the curve depends on the variance; as the variance increases, the curve becomes wider.

When data is distributed normally:

- 68% of values fall in the range: mean −1SD to mean +1SD
- 96% of values fall in the range: mean −2SD to mean +2SD
- 99% of values fall in the range: mean −3SD to mean +3SD

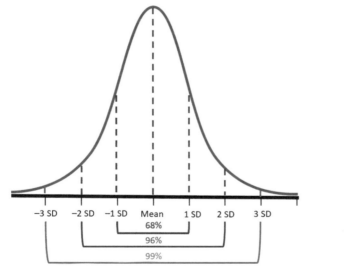

Figure 3.6. Normal distribution curve.

Pragmatically, 95% of data is considered to fall within 2 SD of the mean (rounded from 96%). This distribution range is commonly used to arbitrarily represent the 'normal range'. When values fall outside of this range, they are reported as abnormal. This can be useful in the interpretation of test results and in establishing reference ranges, for example, in the measurement of blood biochemical markers.

Skewed datasets

In some cases, frequency distributions are asymmetrical with a substantially longer tail on one side of the frequency histogram. In these cases, data is termed skewed and the direction of skew depends on the tail.

Positively skewed data has a longer tail on the right. In other words, there are a relatively large number of low values and a lower number of extreme higher values. In positively skewed data, the mean is greater than the median which is greater than the mode.

Negatively skewed data has a longer tail on the left. In other words, there are a relatively large number of high values and a lower number of extreme low values. In negatively skewed data, the mode is greater than the median which is greater than the mean.

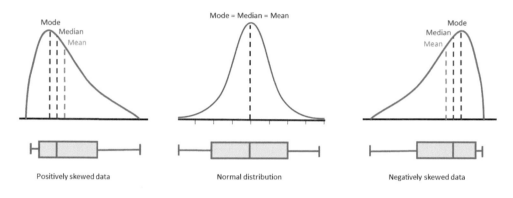

Figure 3.7. Skewed datasets versus the normal distribution.

The t *distribution*

The **t distribution** is a probability distribution that is widely used in statistics. It is most commonly used in studies with a small sample size, usually under 30, and when the population standard deviation is unknown. The *t* distribution looks very similar to the normal distribution curve but shorter and wider, reflecting a greater degree of uncertainty. The exact shape of the *t* distribution is influenced by the mean, variance and degrees of freedom (df) of the data, where df equals the sample size −1.

The *t* distribution has two main applications in statistics:

1. Calculation of the confidence interval (discussed in *Section 3.3.3*)

2. Testing hypotheses about one or more means (discussed in *Section 3.4*).

Figure 3.8 illustrates the *t* distribution. As the sample size increases, the *t* distribution approaches the normal distribution curve. When the sample size is greater than 30, the *t* distribution is very similar to the normal distribution.

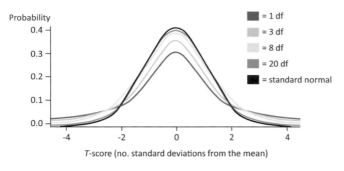

Figure 3.8. The *t* distribution with increasing sample size. As the sample size increases, the *t* distribution approaches the normal distribution.

3.3.2 Standard error of a sample mean

Due to sampling error (discussed in *Section 3.2.2*), the sample estimate varies between different studies and may not always be an accurate representation of the population parameter. For example, imagine that you are interested in estimating the mean HbA1c of all patients with a diagnosis of type 2 diabetes under the care of an endocrine team at a tertiary hospital. In order to do this, you decide to measure the mean HbA1c in a sample of diabetic patients. If this process was repeated 100 times, 100 different sample estimates would be derived and a histogram of these estimates could be plotted. This distribution represents the sampling distribution of the mean. *Figure 3.9* demonstrates the relationship between the frequency distribution for the population parameter and the sampling distribution of the mean in studies with different sample sizes (sample

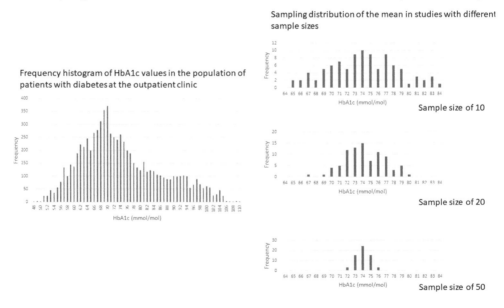

Figure 3.9. Histograms showing the relationship between the frequency distribution of the population parameter and the sampling distribution of the mean. As the sample size increases, the sampling distribution of the mean narrows and the sample estimates become a more precise representation of the population mean.

sizes of 10, 20 or 50). In this example, when the sample size is 10, the range of the sample estimates of HbA1c value is large and ranges from 65mmol/L to 84mmol/L. When the sample size is large, the sample estimates lie closer to the true population mean HbA1c value and the range of estimates decreases. When the sample size is greater than 30, the estimates of the mean follow a normal distribution.

Statistically, the difference between the sample estimate and the population parameter is quantified using the **standard error of the mean (SEM)**. The smaller the SEM, the greater the precision of the sample estimate.

Mathematically, the SEM is calculated using the following formula:

SEM = standard deviation / square root of the sample size

As illustrated in the mathematical formula above, the SEM is influenced by two factors: the standard deviation of the sample estimates and the size of the sample. By increasing the study sample size, the SEM decreases and the sample estimate is more precise. Precision also increases when the sample variance decreases.

3.3.3 Confidence intervals

A research study allows us to calculate a point estimate of the population parameter of interest. Whilst the SEM represents the precision of the estimate, it is not intuitive or easily interpretable by most clinicians. Therefore, the SEM is generally used to estimate the **confidence interval (CI)** for the parameter.

The CI gives a range in which the true population parameter is likely to lie. Most commonly, the 95% confidence interval is used. This is the interval around the sample estimate in which there is a 95% probability that the population parameter lies.

The 95% confidence interval can be calculated using two main methods:

Method 1: Calculation using the normal distribution

As discussed in *Section 3.3.2*, provided that the sample size is large, the sample means follow a normal distribution around the population parametric. We also know that in a normal distribution, approximately 95% of values fall within 1.96 SD of the mean (as discussed in *Section 3.3.1*). When referring to sample estimates in relation to the population parameter, the SD is termed the SEM.

Therefore, in order to calculate the 95% confidence interval, we can apply the following formula:

95% CI = *from* **sample mean − (1.96 × SEM)** *to* **sample mean + (1.96 × SEM)**

Method 2: Calculation using the *t* distribution

Strictly speaking, we should only use Method 1 when the variance in the population is known.

Moreover, Method 1 should only be used when the data is normally distributed. This might not be the case when the sample is small.

If it is not appropriate to use Method 1, we can calculate the confidence interval using the *t* distribution:

95% CI = *from* **sample mean − (**$t_{0.05}$ × **SEM)** *to* **sample mean + (**$t_{0.05}$ × **SEM)**

where $t_{0.05}$ is obtained from a *t* distribution table which can be found online or in a statistics textbook. In order to find the relevant value for $t_{0.05}$, we simply need to reference the value corresponding to the study's degrees of freedom and the desired significance levels. We will talk about this in more detail in *Section 3.4*.

Interpretation of the confidence interval

Consider the following example. In this study, investigators measured the mean change in blood pressure in study participants prescribed a trial medication versus placebo. *Figure 3.10* visualises their results, with the sample estimate represented by the circles and the 95% confidence interval represented by the horizontal lines.

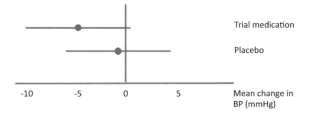

Figure 3.10. A visual representation of sample estimates and confidence intervals. In this example, investigators measured the mean change in blood pressure in study participants prescribed a trial medication versus placebo.

The CI gives us three useful pieces of information:

1. The **width of the confidence interval** represents the precision of the sample estimate. The wider the confidence interval, the less precise and greater the uncertainty of the estimate. In this example, the confidence interval for the trial medication and for the placebo are both around 10mmHg. This suggests that there is a large degree of uncertainty in the estimates for both medications.

2. The **range of the confidence interval** quantifies the magnitude of the effect of interest and enables us to assess the clinical implications of the result. In this example, the effect of the trial medication can be anywhere between a reduction in blood pressure of 10mmHg versus an increase in blood pressure of 1mmHg.

3. The **position of the confidence interval** relative to values of interest, most notably the line of null effect (the value at which there is no association between exposure and outcome or no difference between interventions on outcome). In this example, the confidence interval for the trial medication crosses zero; this suggests that the treatment may not have any effect on blood pressure. This result is commonly extrapolated to suggest that there is no effect of treatment with a significance level of 0.05 (discussed in *Section 3.4.2*).

WORKED EXAMPLE
Hemodynamic effects of sacubitril/valsartan in patients with reduced left ventricular ejection fraction over 24 months: a retrospective study

Abumayyaleh *et al.* (2022) *Am J Cardiovasc Drugs*, **22**: 535, doi.org/10.1007/s40256-022-00525-w

This study aimed to characterise the haemodynamic effects of sacubitril/valsartan in patients with heart failure. In patients who responded to this medication, the risk factors for mortality were investigated. *Table 3.1* summarises the effect of three of the hypothesised predictors of mortality.

Table 3.1: The effect of type 2 diabetes mellitus, congestion at admission and coronary artery disease on mortality

	HR	95% CI	*P* value
Type 2 diabetes mellitus	2.17	0.59–7.92	0.24
Congestion at admission	5.57	1.45–21.48	0.01
Coronary artery disease	3.70	0.47–29.44	0.22

The first column summarises the hazard ratio (HR) corresponding to the three hypothesised predictor variables. As discussed in *Chapter 2*, a HR >1 indicates that the predictor is associated with the outcome. As all three comorbidities have a HR greater than 1, they are all associated with an increased risk of mortality in this cohort. The size of the HR gives us an estimate of the increase in risk. For example, in this study, patients with type 2 diabetes are at 2.17 times greater risk of death than those without. Although this sounds very significant, we need to review the confidence interval before interpreting the significance of these results.

The second column summarises the 95% CI for each of the comorbidities. We can draw the following conclusions from these values:

1. The CI intervals for all three comorbidities are very wide. This indicates low precision of the estimates and a large degree of uncertainty regarding the true HR for the population. To illustrate this further, consider the 95% CI for type 2 diabetes. We can state that we are 95% confident that the true value for HR falls between the range of 0.59 and 7.92. In other words, the true HR could be as low as 0.59 (i.e. protective against death) or as high as 7.92 (i.e. a significant risk factor for death). In this scenario, the large degree of uncertainty makes it difficult to draw any useful conclusions.

2. The CI intervals for type 2 diabetes and coronary artery disease cross the line of null effect (i.e. HR = 1). This is often used as a marker of statistical significance and when this line is crossed, it is often inferred that there is no significant association between the exposure and outcome of interest. Accordingly, in this example, both type 2 diabetes and coronary artery disease are not significantly associated with mortality. This is also represented by the *P* value of greater than 0.05. In contrast, congestion at admission is significantly associated with mortality. This is represented by a 95% confidence interval that does not cross a HR of 1 and a *P* value of 0.01. The interpretation of the *P* value is discussed in detail in *Section 3.4.2*.

3.4   Statistical hypothesis testing and significance levels

Statistical hypothesis testing is a vital concept in medical research. In order to perform statistical hypothesis testing, five main steps need to be performed:

1. Define the **null and alternative hypotheses**.

2. Choose an appropriate **test statistic**.

3. Determine the **critical value of the test statistic**; i.e. at what value do we consider the hypothesis proved or disproved? This is also known as the **significance level**.

4. Perform the statistical test and obtain the *P* value.

5. Interpret the *P* value.

Throughout the next sections of the chapter, we will discuss these steps in more detail.

3.4.1 The null hypothesis

A hypothesis is a proposed explanation for an observation and is the starting point for all clinical research. It is important to define a hypothesis prior to a clinical study taking place. This usually takes the form of the null and alternative hypotheses.

The **null hypothesis (H_0)** states that there is no difference in the outcome of interest between the defined groups.

The **alternative hypothesis (H_1)** states that there is a difference in outcome of interest between groups; this difference can be in either direction (if the hypothesis is two-tailed). One-tailed hypotheses state the direction of effect.

For example, in the ARISTOTLE trial (see *Section 2.10.9*), the null and alternative hypotheses are as follows:

H_0: There is no difference between the risk of ischaemic stroke in patients with AF on warfarin as compared to patients on apixaban.

H_1: There is a difference between the risk of ischaemic stroke in patients with AF on warfarin as compared to patients on apixaban (this could either be increased or decreased risk of stroke).

3.4.2 Significance levels and test statistics

The level of significance should be defined prior to the statistical test being performed. When defined at this stage, it is known as the **alpha value**. The alpha value is the probability of incorrectly rejecting the null hypothesis when it is actually true, i.e. finding a difference due to chance when there is in fact no difference. A value of 0.05 is conventionally chosen. This equates to a 5% chance of incorrectly rejecting the null hypothesis due to the effects of chance.

The ***P* value** is reported after the statistical test has been performed. It is defined as the probability of obtaining the result, or something more extreme, if the null hypothesis is true. In similarity to the alpha value, a P value of 0.05 is conventionally chosen for statistical significance. When the P value is less than 0.05, there is a less than 5% probability that the null hypothesis is true, and therefore we reject the null hypothesis and accept the alternative hypothesis. As the P value approaches zero, there is decreasing evidence in favour of the null hypothesis.

Test statistics

The test statistic describes how closely the distribution of your data matches the distribution predicted under the null hypothesis you are using. The most commonly used test statistics include the Z-score and the T-score. Other test statistics include the f statistic in ANOVA and the chi-square statistic in chi-squared (χ^2) test.

1. The **Z-score** describes the relationship of the mean of the dataset to the mean of the population. It is measured in terms of standard deviation from the population mean. The Z-score ranges from −3 to +3. When the Z-score is 0, it equals the population mean. When it is 1, it is 1 SD from the population mean. Z-scores can be positive or negative depending on whether the value is greater or lower than the mean.

   Mathematically, the Z-score is calculated using the following formula:

$$Z = (X-\mu) / (s/ \sqrt{n})$$

   Where:
   X = sample mean
   μ = population mean
   s = SD of the population means
   n = sample size

2. The **T-score** is similar to the Z-score but is used when the sample size is small and therefore the population mean is not known. The T-score is used in hypothesis testing, using the student's t test (see *Section 3.5.1*).

   Mathematically, the T-score is calculated using the following formula:

$$T = (X - \mu)/ (s/ \sqrt{n})$$

   Where:
   X = sample mean
   μ = population mean
   s = SD of the sample means
   n = sample size

The T-score is traditionally referenced from a t distribution table. In order to look it up, you need to calculate the **degrees of freedom (df)** for your study. The df is dependent on the sample size of the study; the larger the sample size, the greater the df. Using the df, significance level and number of tails, the T-score can be easily referenced in a t distribution table – this can be found online or in any statistics textbook. In practice, T- and Z-scores are always calculated using statistical programs such as SPSS or Excel.

Degrees of freedom (df)

The degrees of freedom of an estimate is the number of independent variables in a dataset. In order to obtain the degrees of freedom for a sample estimate, subtract 1 from the number of measurements. For example, imagine that you are estimating the mean blood pressure reduction with a new medication. If you use 10 people, the df is 9 and if you use 200 people, the df is 199. When calculating df using more than 1 sample from each patient or ANOVA tests, different formulae need to be used.

Once the test statistic has been generated, we can consider its location on the normal or *t* distribution curve. The central region of the curve is the acceptance region. When the test statistic falls within this region, we can infer that there is no statistically significant difference between the sample estimate and the population parameter and we will accept the null hypothesis. The tail(s) of the *t* distribution are the rejection regions. Mostly commonly, both tails are used as rejection regions; this is the case in two-tailed significance tests. Conversely, in one-tailed significance testing, only one tail is used as the rejection area. Hence the hypothesis predicts the direction of effect. In either case, when the sample estimate falls within these areas, we infer that there is a **statistically significant** difference between the sample estimate and population parameter and we reject the null hypothesis. Traditionally, a cut-off value of 1.96 is used for the rejection region; this equates to a significance level of 5%. Statistical tests are used to derive a *P* value from a test statistic. The choice of statistical test is determined by the type of data. This is discussed in *Sections 3.5* and *3.6*.

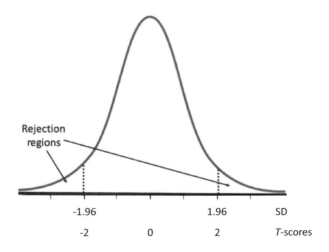

Figure 3.11. Rejection regions on a normal or t distribution curve. In this example, the rejection regions are two-tailed with a significance level of 0.05.

3.4.3 **Types of error (type I versus type II)**

There are two main types of error that occur in hypothesis testing.

A **type I error** occurs when a significant difference between groups is reported when in reality, one does not exist. This is a false positive result, e.g. reporting that an antihypertensive is superior to placebo in lowering blood pressure when in reality there is no difference. Mathematically, the alpha value is the probability of obtaining a type I error. A type I error is more likely to occur in studies with a small sample size due to increased effect of confounding.

A **type II error** occurs when it is incorrectly reported that there is no difference between the two groups when in reality one exists. This is a false negative result, e.g. reporting that an antihypertensive medication does not lower blood pressure when in reality it does. Mathematically, the probability of a type II error is denoted as the **beta value**. Type II errors are more likely to occur when the sample size is small and the study is not powered to detect clinically significant differences between the two groups.

3.4.4 Statistical power

Statistical power is defined as the probability of rejecting the null hypothesis when it is false. It is defined mathematically as 1 – beta. Increased statistical power is associated with a reduced chance of incorrectly failing to reject the null hypothesis, i.e. obtaining a false negative result. In most studies, a power of 80–90% is chosen (this represents 10–20% chance of incorrectly rejecting the null hypothesis).

The power of the study is affected by four major components:

1. Sample size

As sample size increases, power increases.

2. Effect size

The larger the effect size of the treatment, the easier it will be to detect a difference between treatment arms and the larger the power.

3. The variability of the observations

As the variability of the observations increases, the power decreases.

4. Significance level

The larger the significance level, the greater the power of the study but the larger the probability of making a type II error.

In order to increase the power of the study, a larger sample size is generally required. In addition to being more expensive, resource-intensive and time-consuming, recruiting a larger sample may be unethical as more participants are unnecessarily recruited to an experimental study (discussed in *Chapter 4*). Therefore, prior to performing the study, a sample size estimation should be performed. This is an estimation that calculates the sample size required to detect a clinically significant difference. The considerations needed when performing a sample size estimation are summarised in *Section 3.9*.

3.4.5 Multiple hypothesis testing and adjustment

In some studies, multiple hypotheses are tested using the same sample. As the number of hypotheses tested increases, the chance of a type I error increases dramatically. This creates issues with data interpretation and deciding whether a result is truly significant or not. For example, imagine that you are testing 20 different hypotheses in one sample, each with a significance level of 0.05. Mathematically, the probability of obtaining a significant result through the effects of chance alone is equal to $1 - ((1-0.05)^{20})$. This equates to a **64%** chance of observing at least one statistically significant result.

In order to deal with multiple hypothesis testing, the alpha value (the predetermined significance level) can be adjusted. The Bonferroni correction is the simplest adjustment method and adjusts the alpha value dependent on the number of hypotheses tested. It is calculated using the following formula:

Alpha / number of hypotheses tested

The Bonferroni correction assumes that all hypotheses are independent of each other. In research settings, this is often not the case and, in some circumstances, can be overly conservative and result in a very high rate of false negative results.

WORKED EXAMPLE

Efficacy and safety of tofacitinib monotherapy, tofacitinib with methotrexate, and adalimumab with methotrexate in patients with rheumatoid arthritis (ORAL Strategy): a phase 3b/4, double-blind, head-to-head, randomised controlled trial

Fleischmann *et al.* (2017) *Lancet*, 390: 457, doi.org/10.1016/S0140-6736(17)31618-5

The ORAL Strategy study was a phase 3b/4 RCT investigating the efficacy of tofacitinib (a janus kinase inhibitor) compared to adalimumab (an anti-TNF biologic) for the treatment of patients with RA. In this study, participants were randomised to one of three arms; tofacitinib monotherapy (A), tofacitinib with methotrexate (B) or adalimumab with methotrexate (C).

In a two-armed trial, there is only one comparison (A vs. B). In this study, there were three study arms and hence three comparisons (A vs. B, B vs. C, A vs. C). As the number of comparisons increase, the probability of obtaining a false positive result (i.e. a type I error) increases. Some studies, including this example, use a Bonferroni correction to account for this.

In this example, the study investigators used three study arms and hence three comparisons. Therefore, an alpha value of 0.0167 (0.05/3) was used to preserve the overall type I error rate to 5%.

The Bonferroni correction can be used for studies where multiple comparisons are used. These most commonly include studies with more than two treatment arms and studies with multiple endpoints. There is some debate as to when a Bonferroni correction should be used and concern that it increases the risk of false negative results (type II error).

3.5 Statistical significance tests to compare means

In order to choose an appropriate statistical test to compare the means of samples, we need to ask ourselves the following questions.

1. Is the data continuous?

This is a necessity for all of the following statistical tests. Categorical data will be discussed in the next section.

2. How many groups do I want to compare?

3. Is the outcome data parametric or non-parametric?

Parametric statistics are based on assumptions about the population from which the sample was taken. In order to use parametric statistics, the population distribution frequency should follow a normal distribution. Furthermore, the variances in each group should be equal.

Non-parametric statistics are not based on assumptions and this data can be collected from a sample that does not follow the normal distribution.

4. Are the comparison groups independent or dependent?

In independent samples, information about subjects in one group does not provide information about the subjects in the other groups. In this scenario, groups contain different subjects and there is no meaningful way to compare them.

In dependent samples, subjects in one group provide information about other groups. This occurs in two scenarios:

- Measurements are taken from the same individuals at two different time points; for example, before and after an intervention. This is the most common example.

- Measurements are taken from different subjects who have been intentionally matched to each other. For example, in case–control studies, cases and controls may have been matched on the basis of demographic or clinical features. Although the matched pairs are different people, the statistical analysis treats them as the same subject because they are intentionally very similar.

3.5.1 **Selecting a statistical test to compare means**

The following flowchart (*Fig. 3.12*) can be used to identify which statistical test is most appropriate for comparing means.

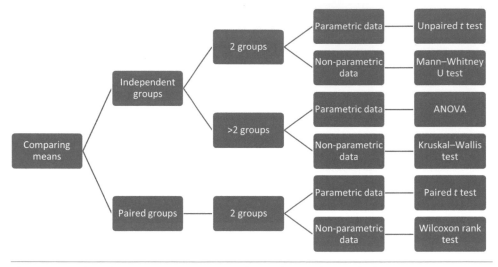

Figure 3.12. Flowchart summarising statistical tests that can be used when comparing means.

After the appropriate test has been chosen, statistical programs such as SPSS or GraphPad can be used to calculate *P* values.

3.6 Statistical significance tests to compare percentages or proportions

In order to choose an appropriate statistical test to compare differences between proportions or percentages between populations, we need to ask ourselves the following:

1. Is the data categorical? (This is a necessity for all of the following statistical tests).

2. How many groups do I want to compare?

3. Are the groups paired or independent?

4. Does the data fulfil the prerequisites required for the statistical test of note?

3.6.1 **Selecting a statistical test to compare percentages**

The following flowchart (*Fig. 3.13*) can be used to identify which statistical test is most appropriate for comparing percentages.

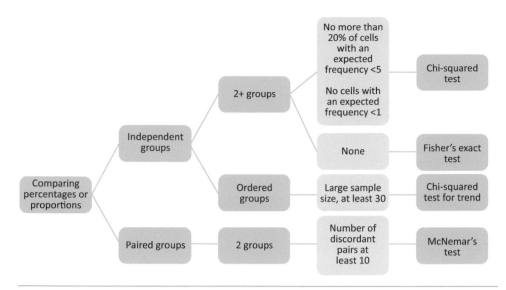

Figure 3.13. Flowchart on statistical tests that can be used when comparing percentages or proportions. Prerequisites are shown in the pink boxes.

WORKED EXAMPLE
Adalimumab reduces extraintestinal manifestations in patients with Crohn's disease: a pooled analysis of 11 clinical studies

Louis *et al.* (2018) *Advances in Therapy*, 35: 563, doi.org/10.1007/s12325-018-0678-0

Background

Extra-intestinal manifestations (EIM) are common in patients with Crohn's disease. This study aimed to investigate the effect of the biological medication adalimumab on EIM in patients with Crohn's disease.

Methods

In order to compare the differences in EIM between the two groups, the authors first described the demographics of recruited subjects and used statistical testing to determine whether there was any difference between the two groups. This is an important part of any study comparing two groups of patients and will be the focus of this worked example.

T tests were used to compare the differences between groups in continuous variables. These included age, disease duration and biochemical markers such as CRP. In this example, the *t* tests are unpaired because the values in one group do not influence the readings in the other. By choosing the *t* test, the authors are assuming that the data is parametric.

Chi-squared tests were used to compare differences between groups in categorical variables including gender and disease activity. By choosing the chi-squared tests, the authors assumed that the data fulfilled the prerequisites outlined in *Figure 3.13*. Data must be independent and must fulfil the expected frequencies requirement when recorded in a two-way table. In this example, a two-way frequency table for gender would appear as follows:

	Male	Female
Adalimumab group	390	747
Placebo group	101	196

In order to perform a chi-squared test, no more than 20% of cells should have an expected frequency of less than five and no cells should have an expected frequency of less than 1.

Results

Table 3.2: A comparison of demographic and disease features in patients in the study on placebo versus adalimumab

	Patients with EIM at baseline		
Characteristic	Placebo (n = 297)	Adalimumab (n = 1137)	P value
Age, years, mean (SD)	38.9 (11.9)	37.5 (12.2)	0.090
Female, n (%)	196 (66.0)	747 (65.7)	0.924
Disease duration, years, mean (SD)	11.0 (8.8)	10.3 (8.5)	
Disease activity			0.001
Moderate, n (%)	149 (50.2)	686 (60.3)	
Severe, n (%)	148 (49.8)	450 (39.6)	
Albumin, g/L, mean (SD)	39.6 (4.8)	39.7 (5.0)	0.701
CRP, mg/dl, mean (SD)	1.7 (2.7)	1.9 (2.7)	0.248

Summary data abstracted from *Advances in Therapy*, 35: 563.

Table 3.2 allows us to compare the two groups and make several conclusions:

1. The patients in the two groups are similar with regard to age, gender, disease duration, albumin level and CRP. This is demonstrated by a P value of greater than 0.05, indicating no difference between the two groups.

2. The patients allocated to receive placebo had higher rates of severe disease activity, compared to those allocated to receive adalimumab. This is demonstrated by a P value of 0.001.

Discussion

This study investigated the difference in EIM in patients with Crohn's disease on adalimumab versus placebo. In order to draw meaningful conclusions, the authors first described the demographic characteristics in the two groups. They used null hypothesis testing to do so and found that the patients allocated to placebo were significantly more likely to have severe disease. This indicates that the two groups are not well matched with respect to disease activity and this could have influenced the overall results from the study. This example describes the use of null hypothesis statistical testing to describe the differences between two groups and indicates the importance of doing this.

3.7   Measures of risk

3.7.1 Relative risk versus odds ratio

In *Chapter 2*, we discussed the calculation of relative risk and odds ratio. A summary of the differences between the two measures is illustrated in *Table 3.3*.

Table 3.3: **A comparison of relative risk versus odds ratio**

	Relative risk	Odds ratio
Definition	Risk in exposed / risk in unexposed	Odds in exposed / odds in unexposed
Measure	Risk = the total number of outcomes in a group divided by the number of people in the group	Odds = the number of outcomes in a group divided by the number of people in the group that did not experience the outcome
Use	Used in a variety of studies including observational studies such as cohort studies and interventional studies such as RCTs	Used in case–control studies; in such cases, the relative risk cannot be used
Interpretation	RR/OR >1: the probability of the outcome occurring is greater in the exposed than the unexposed group	
	RR/OR = 1: the probability of an outcome occurring is the same in the exposed and unexposed groups	
	RR/OR <1: the probability of an outcome occurring is less in the exposed than the unexposed group	
Association	OR approximately equal to RR when outcome is rare	
	OR greater than the RR when the outcome is common	

3.7.2 Absolute risk reduction and number needed to treat

The **absolute risk reduction (ARR)** is another method to compare the risk of an outcome in one group to another. It is calculated using the following equation:

$$\text{ARR} = \text{risk in exposed} - \text{risk in unexposed}$$

The **number needed to treat (NNT)** is derived from the ARR. It is derived from the following calculation:

$$\text{NNT} = 1/\text{ARR}$$

The NNT is the number of patients needed to treat to prevent one adverse outcome (for example; death, heart attack or stroke). It is a measure that is commonly used to report the findings from RCTs and gives a measure of the benefit obtained from a treatment or intervention. The higher the NNT, the more patients need to receive treatment for any benefit to be seen. This information can be used when considering the risk:benefit ratio of a treatment for an individual patient. On a wider level, the NNT gives us an idea of the cost-effectiveness of a treatment.

For example, in classical studies comparing thrombolysis to streptokinase for the management of stroke in the 1980s, there was a 1% ARR in patients treated with thrombolysis. Therefore, 100 patients needed to be treated with thrombolysis for a single patient to gain benefit. At a time when thrombolysis was very expensive, this benefit was not cost-effective and therefore, streptokinase remained the treatment of choice until stronger evidence was reported.

WORKED EXAMPLE
Tocilizumab in patients admitted to hospital with COVID-19 (RECOVERY): a randomised, controlled, open-label, platform trial

RECOVERY Collaborative Group (2021) *Lancet*, **397**: 1637, doi.org/10.1016/S0140-6736(21)00676-0

The aim of this study was to evaluate the efficacy and safety of tocilizumab therapy in adult inpatients admitted with severe Covid-19. The primary outcome was 28-day mortality.

In this trial, 2022 patients were randomised to receive tocilizumab whilst 2094 patients received standard-of-care therapy. In total, 631 participants randomised to the tocilizumab group died compared to 729 participants in the standard-of-care therapy group.

Let's consider the different comparisons of risk:

First, we need to calculate the risk of death in the two groups. This can be done by using the simple calculation:

number of events (in this case 28-day mortality) / total number of participants in group

Therefore, the risk of death in the tocilizumab group is: 621/2022 = **31%**

And the risk of death in the standard-of-care therapy group is: 729/2094 = **35%**

The relative risk is calculated by dividing the risk of death in the treatment group by the risk of death in the standard-of-care therapy group:

$$RR = 31/35 = \mathbf{0.89}$$

As the RR is less than 1, participants receiving tocilizumab had a lower risk of death than those who didn't. This is a proportional measure of risk reduction, in contrast to the ARR which can be calculated as follows:

$$ARR = 35 - 31 = \mathbf{4\%}$$

Therefore, patients receiving tocilizumab had a 4% lower risk of dying than those who didn't. This means that if 100 patients received tocilizumab, four patients would be prevented from dying. This can also be expressed as the NNT:

$$NNT = 1/ARR = 1/0.04 = \mathbf{25}$$

This means that 25 patients need to be treated with tocilizumab in order to prevent one death.

Overall, this data provided strong evidence for the survival benefit with tocilizumab in hospitalised Covid-19 patients.

3.8   Correlation and regression

3.8.1 Introduction

Correlation and regression are used to characterise the relationship between two variables. Correlation allows us to characterise the strength of the association between the two variables and can be used when neither variable is assumed to predict the other. In contrast, regression analyses are used to predict the effect of an explanatory variable on the outcome variable. These analyses can therefore only be used when one variable is thought to change the other.

3.8.2 Correlation

Correlation is a statistical technique used to measure the strength of the association between two variables. There are two main measures of correlation: Pearson correlation coefficient and Spearman correlation coefficient.

Pearson correlation coefficient (r) provides a measure of the correlation between two variables when the relationship between the two is linear. It is a parametric test that can be used when data is normally distributed. r can be calculated using most statistical programs with the result ranging from -1 to $+1$:

1. If r is positive, an increase in one variable results in an increase in the other.

2. If r is negative, an increase in one variable results in a decrease in the other.

3. The magnitude of r indicates how closely the data points lie in relation to the line of best fit. When r is +1 or −1, there is perfect correlation between the two variables.

4. r^2 represents the proportion of the variability in the dependent variable that can be explained by variability in the explanatory variable.

This is graphically depicted in *Figure 3.14*.

Spearman correlation coefficient is a non-parametric measure of correlation. It should be used if any of the following are true, in which cases, it is not possible to perform Pearson correlation.

- The sample size is small
- The relationship between the two variables is non-linear
- Neither x or y are normally distributed.

The value for Spearman correlation coefficient can be interpreted in a similar manner to Pearson correlation coefficient, with a value of +1 or −1 indicating perfect correlation and 0 indicating no correlation.

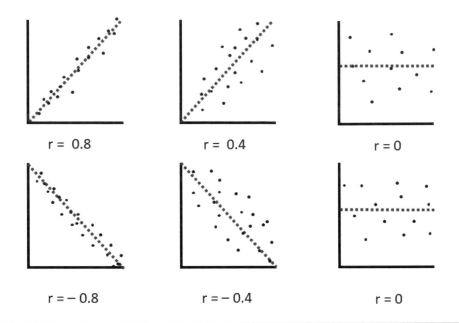

Figure 3.14. Scatter plots demonstrating positive and negative correlation with estimated *r* values.

3.8.3 **Linear regression**

Linear regression quantifies the linear relationship between two continuous variables; an explanatory or independent variable and a dependent variable. In these models, the **explanatory variable** is used to predict the dependent variable.

Imagine a simple study where investigators wanted to determine whether height (explanatory variable) predicts weight (dependent variable) in a cohort of children. In order to do this, the researchers measure the height and weight of 100 children. The next step would involve plotting the results on a scatter graph where *x* is the explanatory variable (height) and *y* is the dependent variable (weight). When the points form a linear relationship, we can plot the regression line; this is the line that best fits through all of the data points (*Figure 3.15*).

The following equation models the simple linear regression line:

$$y = a + bx$$

x = explanatory or independent variable e.g. height (cm)

y = dependent variable e.g. weight (kg)

a = Y intercept of the line

b = the gradient of the line, i.e. how much *y* increases for every unit increase in *x* and in this example, how much weight increases for every centimetre increase in height.

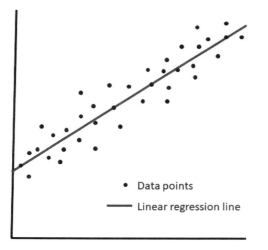

Figure 3.15. Linear regression line.

By plotting the line of best fit, simple linear regression allows us to quantify the values for a and b. This allows us to predict the value of the dependent variable (e.g. weight) for any given value of the explanatory value (e.g. height).

Now that we have discussed the interpretation of the regression line, we can consider methods used for its derivation; most commonly, the method of least squares.

The method of least squares minimises the differences between the observed values and the values predicted by the linear regression line.

Figure 3.16 illustrates the principles of this. Every observed value deviates from the linear regression line. The difference between the observed value and the line is called the residual. The method of least squares minimises the sum of the squares of these residuals, allowing the line to pass through the data points as closely as possible.

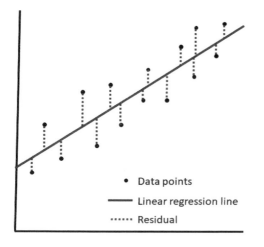

Figure 3.16. Principles of linear regression using the method of least squares.

Assessing goodness of fit

In order to judge how well the line fits the data, we can calculate R^2. This is defined as the percentage of variability of y that can be explained by variability in x. in general, the closer the points lie to the regression line, the higher the value for R^2.

Linear regression is a useful tool to model the association between two continuous variables; however, it can only be performed when the following assumptions are met:

1. There is a linear relationship between x and y.

2. The observations in the sample are independent of each other.

3. The residuals are normally distributed.

4. The residuals have the same variability for all of the fitted values of y.

3.8.4 **Multiple regression**

In some cases, investigators are interested in the effect of several explanatory variables on the dependent variable. Multiple linear regression allows us to investigate this.

Multiple regression allows us to identify whether explanatory variables are associated with the dependent variable. By incorporating more than one explanatory variable into the model, multiple regression allows us to determine the extent to which explanatory variables are associated to the dependent variable after adjusting for other variables (often confounding factors). In similarity to linear regression, multiple regression can allow us to predict the value of the dependent variable from the value of the explanatory variables.

Different regression models are used for different types of explanatory variables.

- Multiple linear regression models include more than one continuous explanatory variable.
- Multiple regression or Analysis of Covariance (ANCOVA) are models with more than one categorical explanatory variable, with or without multiple continuous explanatory variables.

3.8.5 **Logistic regression**

Logistic regression is similar to linear regression except that the dependent variable is a binary outcome; for example, the presence or absence of disease. Like linear regression, logistic regression allows us to characterise which explanatory variables influence the outcome. It can also be used to predict the risk of an outcome in the presence of explanatory variables (usually a risk factor for the development of a disease).

The results from logistic regression are usually presented as odds ratios (OR). In these analyses, both unadjusted and adjusted OR are usually presented. Unadjusted OR represents the association between the explanatory and dependent variable, without taking the other explanatory variables into account. In contrast, the adjusted OR represents the association between the explanatory and dependent variable when all of the explanatory variables are considered. This allows us to consider whether the association between the variables is a true association or whether it is secondary to the presence of confounding variables.

3.8.6 Comparing and contrasting correlation and regression

Table 3.4: Comparing and contrasting correlation and regression

Correlation	Regression
Measures the strength of association between two variables	Describes the effect of the explanatory variable (x) on the dependent variable (y)
The correlation coefficient measures the degree to which two variables move together	Allows us to predict the effect of changes in the explanatory variable on the value of the dependent variables
	Regression analyses quantify the change in the dependent variable for every unit change in the explanatory variable

WORKED EXAMPLE
Dose-response relation between dietary sodium and blood pressure: a meta-regression analysis of 133 randomized controlled trials

Graudal *et al.* (2019) *Am J Clin Nutr*, 109: 1273, doi.org/10.1093/ajcn/nqy384

This study aimed to investigate the effect of reducing sodium intake on blood pressure (BP) measurements in a population of hypertensive individuals. In order to do this, the investigators performed a meta-analysis of 133 RCTs investigating sodium intake on BP. The results from all of the RCTs are plotted in *Figure 3.17* with the size of the circle representing the weight of the individual RCT. In this scatter plot, systolic blood pressure effect is the dependent / y variable and sodium reduction is the explanatory / x variable. A simple linear regression model has been used to characterise the relationship between sodium reduction and BP improvement in patients with a BP greater than 130mmHg.

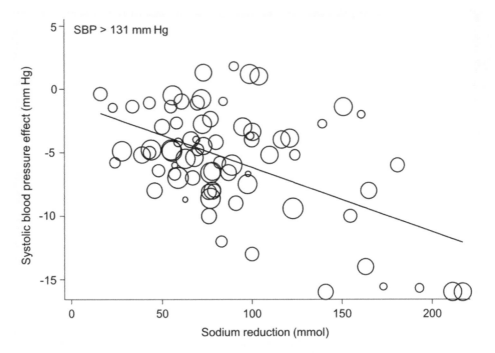

Figure 3.17. Linear regression showing the relationship between systolic blood pressure effect and sodium reduction. Each data point represents a different study, with the size of the circle representative of the size of the study. Reproduced from *Am J Clin Nutr*, 109: 1273 with permission from Oxford University Press.

We can make the following conclusion from these results:

- The gradient of the line represents the improvement in BP for a given reduction in sodium intake. In this case, there is a 5mmHg drop in BP for every 100mmol reduction in sodium intake.

We cannot make the following conclusions:

- Linear regression does not allow us to make predictions about the explanatory variable from the value of the dependent variable. Therefore, we cannot predict the sodium reduction from a patient's SBP.
- We cannot use this model to make predictions for values that fall outside of the measured range. For example, it would be inappropriate to predict the BP effect of reducing sodium intake by 300mmol.
- In this paper, a measure of goodness of fit was not reported. Therefore, we cannot comment on the proportion of variability in BP reduction explained by the sodium reduction.

In this study, the authors went on to perform a multivariable analysis to allow for adjustment of confounding factors. The results from both analyses are summarised in *Table 3.5*.

Table 3.5: Study results from the univariable analysis (simple linear regression model) and the multivariable analysis

Baseline BP	Univariable analysis		Multivariable analysis	
	Effect (95% CI) in mm Hg	*P* value	Effect (95% CI) in mm Hg	*P* value
SBP >131mmHg	−5.0 (−7.1, −3.0)	0.0001	−6.2 (−8.5, −3.9)	0.0001

As previously discussed, in the simple linear model, there was a 5mmHg drop in BP for every 100mmol reduction in sodium intake. This is a statistically significant result with a *P* value of 0.0001. In model 1 of the multivariable analysis, the researchers adjusted for possible confounding factors including baseline BP, age, ethnicity and antihypertensive use. Some of these explanatory variables were continuous (e.g. baseline BP) and others were categorical (e.g. ethnicity). When the multiple regression model was used, a significant impact of sodium reduction on BP improvement remained.

3.9   Determination of sample size

It is essential to perform a sample size calculation during the planning of any confirmatory research study. This determines the number of participants needed to detect a statistically significant difference between the study groups.

3.9.1 Exploratory versus confirmatory research

The differentiation between exploratory and confirmatory research is essential when planning and appraising clinical studies. Broadly speaking, exploratory research aims to generate new hypotheses in areas where little may be known. In contrast, confirmatory research builds upon data from exploratory research in order to test existing hypotheses. The main differences between the two research types are summarised in *Table 3.6*.

Table 3.6: Comparing and contrasting exploratory vs. confirmatory research

Exploratory research	Confirmatory research
Explores unknown research questions	Tests a priori hypotheses
Discovers new knowledge and is not based on previous studies	Generally based on previous studies
Does not offer final and conclusive statements but generates hypotheses to test in confirmatory research	Provides evidence to make inferences from the sample about the population
Less stringent research methods	More stringent research methods
Generates data for sample size calculations in confirmatory research	Sample size calculation should be performed prior to the study
Descriptive statistics and accuracy of sample estimates can be performed	Descriptive statistics and accuracy of sample estimates can be performed
Null hypothesis statistical testing should not be performed	Null hypothesis statistical testing can be performed

3.9.2 Sample size calculations

In order to perform a sample size estimation, the following pieces of information should be considered. It is important to discuss all of these factors with a statistician during the planning of any clinical trial.

- The smallest magnitude of a **clinically significant difference**
  - For example, in a study of antihypertensive medications, we need to consider the fall in blood pressure that would be considered as clinically meaningful. This is based on prior research; for example, the fall in blood pressure required to reduce the risk for cardiovascular outcomes.
- The expected **standard deviation** of observations in each group
  - This is estimated from previous research.
- The **power** that is required of the study
  - Statistical power was discussed in *Section 3.4.4*. The power of the study describes the likelihood that it will detect a clinically significant difference between groups, if one exists in reality.
  - In most studies, the power is set at 80–90%.
- The type of **statistical test** that will be performed with the results
  - When planning a study, it is useful to consider the type of statistical analysis that will be performed with the results. Prior to performing the study, researchers often meet with a statistician to develop a plan for statistical testing that can be added to the study protocol.
- The **critical level of significance** chosen
  - We know that a higher critical level of significance is associated with a decreased risk of type I error (false positive) and increased risk of type II error (false negative).
  - Traditionally, we select a cut significance level of <0.05. At this cut-off level, in 5% of cases, a type II error will be reported.

WORKED EXAMPLE
Efficacy and safety of albendazole and high-dose ivermectin coadministration in school-aged children infected with Trichuris trichiura in Honduras: a randomized controlled trial

Matamoros *et al.* (2021) *Clin Infect Dis*, 73: 1203, doi.org/10.1093/cid/ciab365

The following paragraph has been taken from a study comparing the efficacy of albendazole (ALB) and ivermectin (IVM) in the treatment of parasitic infection in children in Honduras.

Sample size was calculated estimating the efficacy of the different experimental drug or combinations and gathering the individual samples sizes for the study. The sample size was calculated using a 1-tailed test for pairwise comparisons of the expected cure rates for 4 study groups – 17% for single-does ALB, 55% for single-dose ALB-IVM, 85% for 3-dose ALB-IVM, and 60% for 3-dose AL – with an overall significance level of 5% adjusted for multiple tests by Bonferroni correction and 80% power and inflated for 10% loss to follow-up. The estimated sample size was 177 participants, included 39 participants for single-dose ALB (arm 1), 57 for single-dose ALB-IVM (arm 2), 24 for 3-dose ALB (arm 3), and 57 for 3-dose ALB-IVM (arm 4).

As you can see the authors have considered:

1. The statistical test that will be used; in this case, a 1-tailed test for pairwise comparisons.
2. The expected cure rates with the different medications; this data has been taken from the existing literature.
3. The significance level required; the study has followed convention and used a cut-off of 5%.
4. As multiple hypotheses have been tested, the authors corrected the 5% significance level using the Bonferroni correction. This was discussed in *Section 3.4.5*.
5. A power of 80% was selected; this is a common value to use.
6. The number of participants lost to follow-up was estimated to be 10%.

Overall, the sample size calculation estimated that 177 participants would need to be recruited to the study. The authors stuck to this estimation and recruited a total of 176 children to the study. Recruiting more children would be unnecessarily time-consuming and costly.

3.10 Analysis of survival data

Survival analyses characterise the time an individual takes to reach an endpoint of interest, often but not always death.

3.10.1 Kaplan–Meier survival curves

A survival curve is usually calculated by the Kaplan–Meier method and displays the cumulative probability of an individual remaining free of the endpoint of interest at any time after baseline. The cumulative probability will only change once an endpoint has occurred. Therefore, the curve is drawn in a series of steps, starting at a survival probability of 100% and falling towards 0% as time increases.

An example of a survival curve is illustrated in *Figure 3.18*:

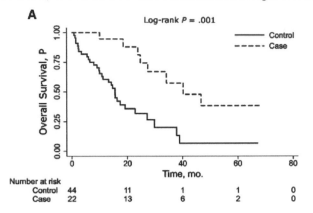

Figure 3.18. Kaplan–Meier curve showing overall survival of patients diagnosed with pancreatic cancer with ATM mutations (cases) and without (controls). Figure reproduced from *JNCI Cancer Spectrum*, 2021: 5: pkaa121, with permission from Oxford University Press.

This study characterised the survival of patients with pancreatic cancer with and without pathogenic mutations in ATM. This Kaplan–Meier curve illustrates survival time following a diagnosis of pancreatic cancer. In this example, the cases did not have pathogenic ATM mutations, whereas the control patients did. As in all survival curves, percentage survival falls with time in a stepwise fashion as events (deaths) occur.

Kaplan–Meier survival curves can be used to generate the following useful pieces of information:

- Survival rates at defined time points
  - This is a common method of explaining survival data, for example, the 1-, 5- or 10-year survival rate.
  - In the above example, the 20-month survival rate is around 85% in cases compared to only around 35% in controls.
- Median survival time (i.e. the time at which 50% of the patients are still alive)
  - In order to determine this, simply note the time at which the survival curve crosses 50%.
  - In the above example, the median survival in cases was 40.2 months compared to 15.5 months in the controls.

In the majority of cases, survival analyses measure an adverse endpoint, usually death. When the endpoint is favourable, such as recovery, the Kaplan–Meier curve is conventionally plotted upwards. In these scenarios, the curve starts at zero and increases towards 100% as time progresses.

3.10.2 Censored data

An important concept in survival analysis is censoring. When a patient's data is censored, this means that we do not know the true survival time for the patient. There are three main reasons for this:

1. The patient does not reach the endpoint by the time that the study has finished.

2. The patient withdraws from the study.

3. The patient is lost to follow-up during the period of the study.

There are two main types of censored data:

Right censored data is the most common. It occurs when the patient does not reach the endpoint during the study. This is either because the patient survives until the end of the study or because they withdraw from the study before they reach the endpoint. In both cases, the exact survival time is not known; however, the true survival time will always be greater than the observed survival time.

In contrast, in **left censored data**, the true survival time is shorter than the observed survival time. This is rare but can occur in some circumstances. For example, imagine measuring the survival time of people infected with hepatitis C. In this scenario, survival time is measured from the date of serological diagnosis. In these cases, it is generally not possible to determine the exact time of infection. As infection precedes diagnosis, observed survival time is shorter than the true survival time.

Censored data is usually plotted as a plus on the survival curve.

3.10.3 **Log rank test**

Statistical methods can be used to compare differences in the survival times in the two groups studied. The log rank test is one such method. This is a non-parametric test that guides the acceptance or rejection of the null hypothesis. The downside of this test is that it cannot assess the independent roles of more than one factor on the time to endpoint, and therefore cannot correct for confounding factors.

3.10.4 **The Cox proportional hazards model and hazard ratios**

The Cox model is the most widely used method to analyse time-to-event data. The model uses regression analysis to provide an estimate of the **hazard ratio**. This is the ratio of hazard rate in one group compared to the hazard rate in another group, where the hazard rate describes the probability of an outcome occurring over a defined time period.

The major advantage of the Cox model is that it can test the effects of explanatory variables on the time-to-endpoint. These variables can take the form of continuous, binary or categorical data. For example, imagine a study investigating the survival of patients following a new chemotherapy agent. The Cox model allows us to investigate whether a range of explanatory variables, such as patient age, sex or cancer stage, affect survival time. Clearly, this gives us important clinical information and allows us to determine which patients are most likely to benefit from this new treatment.

The major disadvantage of the Cox model is that it assumes that the hazard ratio is constant over time. When this is not the case, the Cox model should not be used, at least not in its most simple form.

Interpreting hazard ratios from the Cox model

Interpretation of the hazard ratio is similar to interpretation of the relative risk.

HR = 1 → there is no relationship between the explanatory variable and the outcome of interest.

HR <1 → the explanatory variable is protective against developing the hazard.

HR >1 → the explanatory variable is a risk factor for developing the hazard.

WORKED EXAMPLE
Association between bone mineral density at different anatomical sites and both mortality and fracture risk in patients receiving renal replacement therapy: a longitudinal study

Jaques *et al.* (2022) *Clin Kidney J*, 15: 1188, doi.org/10.1093/ckj/sfac034

This study aimed to investigate the effect of bone mineral density (BMD) on survival and fracture risk in patients with end-stage renal disease on renal replacement therapy (RRT).

Figure 3.19 represents a Kaplan–Meier curve demonstrating the risk of fracture (hip and overall) in patients with low BMD (blue line) compared to high BMD (red line).

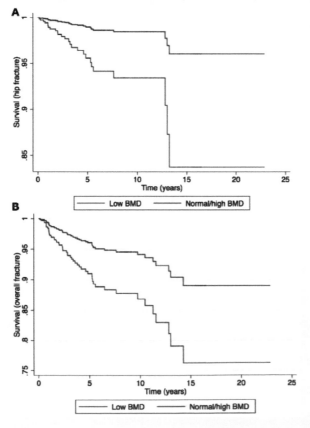

Figure 3.19. Worked example outlining the interpretation of Kaplan–Meier curves. These Kaplan–Meier curves clearly illustrate that patients with a low BMD have increased risk of hip and overall fracture compared to those with normal or high BMD. At 10 years, around 7% of patients with a low BMD have suffered from a hip fracture compared to around 2% of patients with normal or high BMD. Reproduced from *Clin Kidney J*, 15: 1188 with permission from Oxford University Press.

Table 3.7: Table summarising HR (95% CI) and *P* values for hip and any fracture using BMD as a predictor variable (normal/high versus low). In this example, the authors have used three models to assess the risk of BMD on hip and any fracture.

Model	HR (95% CI)	P value
Hip fracture		
Univariate model	0.21 (0.10–0.45)	<0.001
Partially adjusted model	0.33 (0.15–0.74)	0.007
Fully adjusted model	0.22 (0.08–0.62)	0.004
Any fracture		
Univariate model	0.30 (0.18–0.50)	<0.001
Partially adjusted model	0.45 (0.26–0.77)	0.004
Fully adjusted model	0.42 (0.21–0.83)	0.013

As you can see, patients with a normal/high BMD have a HR <1 when compared to those with a low BMD. This suggests that normal/high BMD is protective against fractures (hip and total).

The use of different models in this analysis allows for adjustment for confounding factors. The first model (the univariate model) does not correct for confounding factors. The partially adjusted model corrects for the confounders RRT mode, age and gender. The fully adjusted model corrects for the above confounders in addition to BMI, ethnicity, gender, PTH, smoking and CRP. These are all factors that are known to influence fracture risk. In all three models, the effect of BMD on fracture risk remains significant. Therefore we can conclude that low BMD is associated with increased risk of fracture, even when confounding factors are accounted for.

Conclusion

In conclusion, this study demonstrated that patients on RRT with a low BMD were more likely to suffer from fractures than those with a normal or high BMD.

3.11 Meta-analysis

As discussed in *Section 2.11.3*, a meta-analysis is a type of systematic review that combines numerical data from multiple studies.

3.11.1 Forest plots

A **forest plot** is the most common method to display the results from a meta-analysis (see *Fig. 3.22* for an example). A forest plot summarises the estimated effect from individual trials and a summary measure which is derived from pooling the results from all of the studies.

The solid vertical line in a forest plot represents the 'line of no effect'. This corresponds to a relative risk or odds ratio of one.

The results from individual studies are plotted vertically, with each study graphically represented by a box and a line. The location of the box gives us the effect estimate from the study of note. The size of the box corresponds to the weighting of the study to the summary measure. This is usually dependent on the size of the study, with larger studies carrying more weight and hence represented by larger squares. The length of the horizontal line represents the confidence interval of each study.

The summary measure is usually represented by a diamond. This is the weighted average of the effect estimates from all included studies and gives us the effect estimate from the meta-analysis. The horizontal length of the diamond represents the confidence interval of the summary estimate. The longer the diamond, the less certain we are in the summary result.

3.11.2 **Publication bias**

As discussed in *Chapter 2*, one disadvantage to meta-analysis is publication bias. This describes the tendency for studies with positive results to be published over those with negative results.

To consider whether publication bias is present, we can draw a **funnel plot**. This is a scatter diagram of all published studies with treatment effect on the horizontal axis and a measure of study precision, such as standard error, on the vertical axis.

When there is no publication bias, the funnel plot is symmetrical. If publication bias is present, the funnel is asymmetrical. This is depicted graphically in *Figure 3.20*, where published studies are generally larger or have a larger effect size. By omitting the results from the missing or unpublished studies, the estimated effect size is artificially inflated.

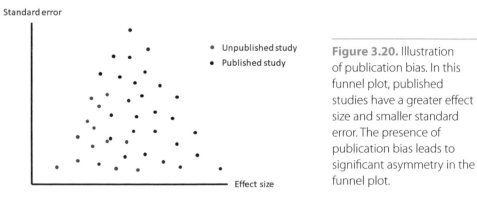

Figure 3.20. Illustration of publication bias. In this funnel plot, published studies have a greater effect size and smaller standard error. The presence of publication bias leads to significant asymmetry in the funnel plot.

If there is significant publication bias, there will be substantial asymmetry on the funnel plot. If the funnel plot appears grossly symmetrical, statistical tests, such as the Begg rank correlation test or Egger linear regression test, can be used to assess for publication bias. These methods should only be used when there are at least ten studies in the meta-analysis, as the power of the test is too low to distinguish chance from real asymmetry. These tests can also be used to adjust for publication bias.

3.11.3 **Tests for heterogeneity**

In the context of meta-analysis, heterogeneity implies differences between study estimates. Heterogeneity occurs due to differences between study protocol, study design and participant demographics or comorbidities.

Statistical methods can be used to test for heterogeneity in meta-analyses. The I^2 statistic is a common measure of heterogeneity. It provides an estimate of the proportion of the total variability between estimates that can be attributed to heterogeneity between studies. The I^2 statistic ranges between 0 and 100. The higher the I^2, the larger the degree of heterogeneity. Although there is no hard and fast rule, we generally consider heterogeneity to be present when the I^2 is greater than 50%. When the I^2 is very large, the validity of combining study results, and therefore the summary estimate, is called into question.

The presence of heterogeneity has multiple implications:

- Researchers use random effects methods rather than fixed effects methods (this is discussed in *Section 2.11.3)*
- Researchers can explore the treatment effects between groups with the aim of finding groups where homogeneity exists. For instance, a treatment may have a beneficial effect in one subgroup compared to another. By identifying this group, we can target the treatment to the right patient cohort.

WORKED EXAMPLE
Statin use and mortality in COVID-19 patients: updated systematic review and meta-analysis

Kollias *et al*. (2021) *Atherosclerosis,* 330: 114, doi.org/10.1016/j.atherosclerosis.2021.06.911

Background

Statins are lipid-lowering medications that are prescribed to patients with high cardiovascular risk. In previous studies, statins have demonstrated cardioprotective and immunomodulatory effects. In light of these effects, observational studies have been performed to investigate whether statins are associated with improved survival in patients with Covid-19. This study performed a systematic review and meta-analysis of observational studies investigating the relationship between statin use and Covid-19-related mortality.

Methods

In this review, 22 studies fulfilled the inclusion criteria and were included in the meta-analysis. Of these studies, 12 studies reported odds ratios and 10 studies reported hazard ratios. We will focus on the studies reporting odds ratio.

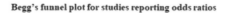

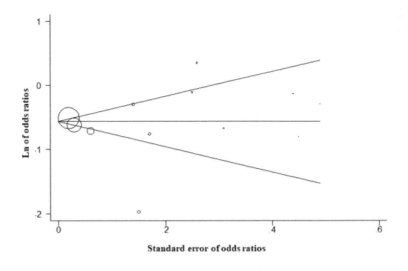

Begg's funnel plot for studies reporting odds ratios

Standard error of odds ratios

Figure 3.21. A worked example of a funnel plot. Reproduced from *Atherosclerosis*, 330: 114 with permission from Elsevier.

The authors used funnel plots to assess for publication bias. In this example, the ln(odds ratio) is plotted on the vertical axis and the standard error of the odds ratio is plotted on the horizontal axis. Each study is represented by an individual circle, with larger circles representing larger studies. In this example, the funnel appears roughly symmetrical; however, its interpretation is limited by a small number of included studies.

Results

The results from the meta-analysis of studies reporting odds ratios are illustrated in *Figure 3.22*. The 12 included studies are listed vertically. As you can see, there are two large studies (Rosenthal and Mallow) that contribute 50% of the weighting to the pooled estimate. These studies are associated with a OR <1, and hence a protective effect of statins on Covid-19-related mortality. The remainder of the studies are smaller and contribute a smaller weighting to the pooled estimate. These studies are represented by small boxes and wide confidence intervals.

The pooled OR estimate is 0.65 with a 95% confidence interval ranging from 0.55 to 0.78. Therefore, we are 95% certain that statin users have a OR of 0.55 to 0.78 for Covid-19-related mortality compared to non-statin users. This is a significant result with a *P* value <0.01 indicating that statin users are significantly less likely to die from Covid-19 than non-users.

In this meta-analysis, heterogeneity is present (I^2 = 61%). This could be explained by between-study differences in statin dose, statin class, patient characteristics or Covid-19 severity. Further work is needed to investigate the cause of heterogeneity and whether certain patients are more likely to benefit from statin therapy.

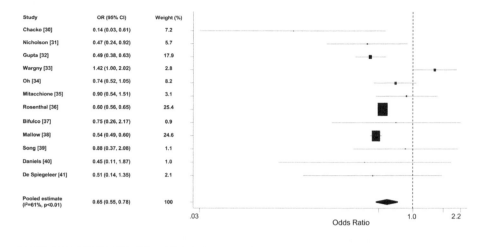

Study	OR (95% CI)	Weight (%)
Chacko [30]	0.14 (0.03, 0.61)	7.2
Nicholson [31]	0.47 (0.24, 0.92)	5.7
Gupta [32]	0.49 (0.38, 0.63)	17.9
Wargny [33]	1.42 (1.00, 2.02)	2.8
Oh [34]	0.74 (0.52, 1.05)	8.2
Mitacchione [35]	0.90 (0.54, 1.51)	3.1
Rosenthal [36]	0.60 (0.56, 0.65)	25.4
Bifulco [37]	0.75 (0.26, 2.17)	0.9
Mallow [38]	0.54 (0.49, 0.60)	24.6
Song [39]	0.88 (0.37, 2.08)	1.1
Daniels [40]	0.45 (0.11, 1.87)	1.0
De Spiegeleer [41]	0.51 (0.14, 1.35)	2.1
Pooled estimate (I^2=61%, p<0.01)	0.65 (0.55, 0.78)	100

Figure 3.22. A worked example of a forest plot. Reproduced from *Atherosclerosis*, 330: 114 with permission from Elsevier.

Conclusion

In conclusion, this meta-analysis suggests that statins are associated with a lower mortality rate in patients with Covid-19. Limitations to this study include its observational and retrospective nature. Furthermore, there was significant heterogeneity between studies, likely due to differences in study protocol, treatment regimen and patient characteristics.

3.12 Diagnostic tests

Together with history taking and clinical examination, investigations are vital in the diagnosis of many clinical conditions. No diagnostic test is 100% accurate in the detection of disease, and this section will discuss the measures of test validity.

3.12.1 Sensitivity and specificity

When evaluating the diagnostic utility of a test, we commonly consider the sensitivity and the specificity of the test.

In order to understand the definition of sensitivity and specificity, consider the following 2×2 table outlining the frequencies of test results in those with and without the disease of interest.

Test result	Disease	No disease
Positive	a	b
Negative	c	d

Specificity = the proportion of individuals without the disease who test negative using the test
= d / b + d

Sensitivity = the proportion of individuals with the disease who test positive using the test
= a / a + c

In an ideal world, all tests would be 100% sensitive and 100% specific for the diagnosis of disease. In clinical practice, tests often gain sensitivity at the expense of specificity and vice versa. Whether we aim for high sensitivity or high specificity depends on the disease in question. For example, tests with a high sensitivity are preferred when the disease of interest is easily treatable. In this scenario, we want to detect all cases of disease in order to provide treatment.

3.12.2 Predictive value

Whilst the sensitivity and specificity of the test characterise the diagnostic ability of the test, the predictive values indicate how likely it is that the individual has the disease in light of their test result.

Positive predictive value (PPV) = proportion of individuals with a positive test who have the disease
= a / (a + b)

Negative predictive value (NPV) = proportion of individuals with a negative test who do not have the disease
= c / (c + d)

The predictive values depend on the prevalence of the disease in the population of interest. In samples where the disease is common, the PPV is higher than in samples where the disease is rare.

3.12.3 Likelihood ratios and pre- and post-test odds

The **likelihood ratio (LR)** gives another measure of the performance of the test. It is calculated using the following formula:

$$LR = sensitivity / (1-specificity)$$

Therefore, when the LR is greater than 1, the test is more likely to give a positive result if the patient has the disease than if they did not. The greater the LR, the greater the discriminatory power of the test.

The pre- and post-test odds are the odds of the patient having the disease before and after the test is performed. Before the test is performed, the odds of the patient having the disease are the same as the general population. This is calculated as:

$$\textbf{Pre-test odds} = prevalence (1-prevalence)$$

Following a positive test result, the odds of disease (post-test odds) depend on both the pre-test odds and the LR of the test. The post-test odds are calculated as:

$$\textbf{Post-test odds} = \text{pre-test odds} \times \text{LR}$$

3.12.4 Receiver operating characteristic (ROC) curves

A ROC curve is used to determine a cut-off value for a diagnostic test, i.e. the value at which we state that the test is positive. The ROC curve is a plot of sensitivity versus (1 − specificity) across different cut-off values. A ROC curve is usually plotted with a line at an angle of 45°; this represents a test that performs no better than chance. The better the discriminatory capacity of the test, the closer the curve lies to the upper left-hand corner. The area under the curve (AUC) summarises the location of the curve, giving a combined measure of the sensitivity and specificity and hence the validity of the test. The higher the AUC, the higher the validity of the test. Mathematically, the AUC represents that a randomly chosen diseased individual is rated as more likely to have the disease by the test. The maximum AUC is 1, meaning that the test perfectly discriminates between diseased and non-diseased individuals. An AUC of 0.5 indicates that the test performs equally to chance. The AUC provides a useful measure of the test performance and allows us to compare the validity of multiple diagnostic tests.

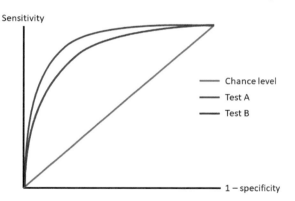

Sensitivity

— Chance level
— Test A
— Test B

1 − specificity

Figure 3.23. Two ROC curves in comparison to chance level. The ROC curve for test A lies closer to the upper left corner of the graph and has a higher AUC and hence validity, as compared to test B.

WORKED EXAMPLE
Diagnostic value of anti-cyclic citrullinated peptide antibody in patients with rheumatoid arthritis

Zeng *et al.* (2003) *J Rheumatol*, 30: 1451, PMID: 12858440.

Background

The detection of anti-cyclic citrullinated peptide (CCP) antibody is a widely used diagnostic test in the investigation of rheumatoid arthritis (RA). This study aimed to describe the validity of a novel ELISA for the measurement of anti-CCP in the diagnosis of RA.

Methods

In this study, the authors described a modified ELISA for the detection of anti-CCP antibodies. In order to describe the sensitivity and specificity of the ELISA, the investigators tested the serum of 191 patients with RA and 230 control subjects (including healthy controls and patients with non-RA rheumatological diagnoses).

Results

Table 3.8: A 2×2 table outlining the frequencies of CCP positivity in those with and without RA

	RA	Control patient
CCP positive	90	6
CCP negative	101	230

Table 3.8 summarises the results from the study. From this data, we can calculate the sensitivity and specificity of the anti-CCP ELISA:

Specificity = the proportion of individuals without the disease who test negative using the test
= 230 / (230 + 6) = 97.4%

As the specificity of the test is high, false positive results are rare (2.6% of all positive results). Therefore, we can conclude that the test is highly specific for RA and a positive result means that the patient is highly likely to have the disease.

Sensitivity = the proportion of individuals with the disease who test positive using the test
= 90 / (90 + 101) = 47.1%

The sensitivity of the test is only 47%. Therefore, only 47% of people with RA test positive for anti-CCP using this ELISA. This means that the test has a high false negative rate and cannot be used to rule out the diagnosis of RA.

The authors calculated the PPV and NPV of the anti-CCP test in the study population. It is important to remember that the PPV and NPV are population-specific. Therefore, these results cannot be extrapolated to the wider population when the prevalence of RA is much lower than the study cohort.

PPV = proportion of individuals with a positive test who have the disease
= 90 / (90 + 6)
= 94%

Therefore, in this population, 94% of patients with a positive test had RA.

NPV = proportion of individuals with a negative test who do not have the disease
= 230 / (230 + 101)
= 69%

Therefore, 69% of patients with a negative test did not have RA.

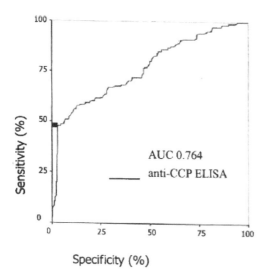

Figure 3.24. A worked example of a ROC curve. Reproduced from the *Journal of Rheumatology* with permission.

The authors plotted a ROC curve to determine the optimal value for the cut-off for a positive result. A cut-off value of 99 units was found to produce the optimal sensitivity and specificity. The AUC equals 0.764.

Conclusion

In this study, the presence of anti-CCP antibodies was highly specific but moderately sensitive for the diagnosis of RA. Therefore, testing for anti-CCP antibody provides a useful adjunct in the diagnosis of RA, but a negative test cannot be used to rule out the diagnosis.

3.13 Chapter summary

Throughout this chapter, we have introduced some of the principles and methods that are commonly used in the statistical analysis of clinical research. Further detail can be found in dedicated statistics textbooks. Given the complexity of the subject, it is always important to include statisticians in the design, undertaking and analysis of research studies.

3.14 Further reading

Statistics at Square One: www.bmj.com/about-bmj/resources-readers/publications/statistics-square-one

Understanding statistics 1: presenting data from clinical trials: https://learning.bmj.com/learning/module-intro/.html?moduleId=5003158

Understanding statistics 2: what is statistical uncertainty?: https://learning.bmj.com/learning/module-intro/.html?moduleId=5001080

Harris, M. and Taylor, G. (2020) *Medical Statistics Made Easy*, 4e. Scion Publishing Ltd.

Peacock, J.L. and Peacock P.J. (2020) *Oxford Handbook of Medical Statistics*, 2e. Oxford University Press.

Petrie, A. and Sabin, C. (2020) *Medical Statistics at a Glance*, 4e. Wiley-Blackwell.

CHAPTER 4

Ethical considerations and governance

4.1 Introduction

Research governance concerns the regulations and standards that ensure research is carried out to a high standard and that the rights and safety of participating individuals are maintained. Ethical considerations play a major role in ensuring high-quality research; high-quality research cannot be unethical! Ethical guidelines therefore play an important role in research governance and the two concepts are closely linked. Throughout this chapter, we will discuss the ethical and governance considerations at each stage of a research study.

4.2 Core ethical values of clinical research

Ethics is an inseparable component of clinical medicine and clinical research. It concerns the moral framework that ensures the safety, wellbeing and autonomy of patients and study participants. Ethics provides guidelines to address moral dilemmas that are commonly encountered in clinical research. The four principles model (see *Table 4.1*) is the most widely used ethical framework and was defined by Beauchamp and Childress in 1979. It defines four key principles in medical ethics: beneficence, non-maleficence, autonomy and justice.

Table 4.1: The four principles model of medical ethics and their application in clinical medicine and clinical research

Principle	Definition	Application in clinical medicine	Additional considerations in clinical research
Beneficence	Healthcare workers have a duty to act in the best interests of the patient	Patients should be treated with effective management that is expected to result in clinical benefit	When available, study participants should be prescribed effective treatments alongside trial medications
Non-maleficence	Healthcare workers have a duty to prevent harm to the patient	Healthcare workers should balance the benefits and harms of the treatment and avoid treatments that are inappropriately burdensome or harmful	Phase 1 studies are considered high risk for participating subjects; therefore, researchers must take all of the necessary steps to minimise the risk of harm
Autonomy	Competent individuals have the right to make their own decisions regarding their healthcare Autonomy includes a right to privacy	Patients must give informed consent regarding their management Healthcare workers have a duty to maintain confidentiality and uphold data protection rules	Informed consent is more rigorous than in clinical medicine and requires written documentation and signed consent forms Participants have a right to withdraw from a study at any time without any reason
Justice	Healthcare workers must respect the rights of individuals On a wider societal level, healthcare resources should be distributed fairly	Patients should not be discriminated against on the basis of factors including age, gender and ethnicity	There should be a fair method of recruiting study participants into the clinical trial Enrolled participants should be treated equally

In addition to these four core pillars of medical ethics, there are many other considerations in clinical research. Some of these principles include:

- Essentiality
  - Prior to a research study being performed, it is vital to review the existing literature to ensure that the study will provide important new information. This should be scrutinised by an independent review, with the conclusion that the research is likely to benefit the public.
- Professional competence
  - Research should only be conducted by individuals with the relevant qualifications and competencies.

- Transparency
  - Research should be conducted in a manner that is fair, honest and impartial. Full and complete records should be retained for a reasonable period following the study for the purpose of post-study monitoring. This can vary based on study requirements.
- Validity
  - Research should be carried out to a high scientific standard to ensure novelty and a useful contribution is made to add to the current literature. If the research process is flawed, the results are unreliable and this undermines the fundamental principles of evidence-based medicine.
- Public domain
  - The results of the study should be brought into the public domain. This is generally done through scientific publication. Where possible, publications should be openly accessible to the public. Through scientific dissemination, this ensures advancement of knowledge in the field, benefiting the public as a whole and preventing unnecessary duplication of studies.

4.3   Ethical guidelines

Humans have experimented on humans for millennia and the history of unethical research dates back to ancient times. Many of the early advances in clinical medicine were achieved at the expense of experimentation on marginalised groups such as prisoners or asylum inmates. The widespread extent of these practices led to calls for formal ethical frameworks in clinical research. Three of these are the Nuremberg Code, the Declaration of Helsinki and Good Clinical Practice.

4.3.1 Nuremberg Code

Following the atrocities that were committed by medical researchers in World War II, the Nuremberg Code (1947) set out ethical guidelines for studies involving experimentation in human subjects. In total, ten research principles were defined. These focused on the human rights of participating study participants. For the first time, the Nuremberg Code outlined an absolute requirement for informed consent in all participating research subjects in addition to the right for subjects to withdraw from participation in a study at any point. The ten standards outlined in the Nuremberg Code can be found at https://media.tghn.org/medialibrary/2011/04/BMJ_No_7070_Volume_313_ The_Nuremberg_Code.pdf.

4.3.2 Declaration of Helsinki

The Declaration of Helsinki (1964) is a statement of ethical principles for medical research involving human subjects that was published by the World Medical Association (WMA). It is an extension of the Nuremberg Code but focuses on the obligations of researchers to participating subjects. The Declaration of Helsinki can be read at https://jamanetwork.com/journals/jama/fullarticle/1760318.

Although neither the Nuremberg Code nor the Declaration of Helsinki are legally binding documents, they have been incorporated into laws that govern research ethics in countries across the world.

4.3.3 Good Clinical Practice

Good Clinical Practice (GCP) is a set of internationally recognised ethical, scientific and practical standards to which all clinical research should be conducted. Compliance with GCP is a legal obligation in many clinical trials and studies.

GCP outlines thirteen key principles that should be followed during clinical research:

1. **Ethics:** clinical trials should be conducted in accordance with the ethical principles that have their origin in the Declaration of Helsinki, and that are consistent with GCP and the applicable regulatory requirement(s).

2. **Trial risk vs. trial benefit:** before a trial is initiated, foreseeable risks and inconveniences should be weighed against the anticipated benefit for the individual trial subject and society. A trial should be initiated and continued only if the anticipated benefits justify the risks.

3. **Trial participants:** the rights, safety and wellbeing of the trial subjects are the most important considerations and should prevail over interests of science and society.

4. **Information on the medicinal product:** the available non-clinical and clinical information on an investigational product should be adequate to support the proposed clinical trial.

5. **Good quality trials:** clinical trials should be scientifically sound, and described in a clear, detailed protocol.

6. **Compliance with the study protocol:** a trial should be conducted in compliance with the protocol that has received prior institutional review board (IRB)/independent ethics committee (IEC) approval/favourable opinion.

7. **Medical decisions:** the medical care given to, and medical decisions made on behalf of, subjects should always be the responsibility of a qualified physician or, when appropriate, of a qualified dentist.

8. **Trial staff:** each individual involved in conducting a trial should be qualified by education, training and experience to perform his or her respective task(s).

9. **Informed consent:** freely given informed consent should be obtained from every subject prior to clinical trial participation.

10. **Clinical trial data:** all clinical trial information should be recorded, handled and stored in a way that allows its accurate reporting, interpretation and verification.

11. **Confidentiality:** the confidentiality of records that could identify subjects should be protected, respecting the privacy and confidentiality rules in accordance with the applicable regulatory requirement(s).

12. **Good manufacturing practice:** investigational products should be manufactured, handled and stored in accordance with applicable good manufacturing practice (GMP). They should be used in accordance with the approved protocol.

13. **Quality assurance**: systems with procedures that assure the quality of every aspect of the trial should be implemented.

GCP training is required for healthcare professionals embarking on clinical research. Free online GCP courses can be accessed through the NIHR Learn platform.

4.4 Ethical and governance processes involved in setting up a study

Before a study can commence, there are many governance and ethical considerations to think about. These will be discussed throughout the next part of the chapter.

4.4.1 Study classification

The first step in setting up a research study is formulating the research question. After this has been done, the study will fall into one of two categories. It is important to consider which category the study falls into, because this dictates the relevant governance protocols and legislation.

1. **Clinical trials of an investigational medicinal product (CTIMPs)** are interventional trials that investigate the efficacy, safety or pharmacodynamics of investigational medicinal products (IMPs; aka medications) in human subjects. They are subject to stricter legislation than non-CTIMPs and must be performed following the guidance set out by the UK Medicines for Human Use (Clinical Trials) Regulations 2004. CTIMPs are regulated by the Medicines and Healthcare products Regulatory Agency (MHRA) and adherence to GCP is a legal requirement for these studies.

2. **Non-CTIMPs** do not involve an **investigational medicinal product (IMP)** and therefore, do not fall into the scope of the Medicines for Human Use (Clinical Trials) Regulations 2004. Many different clinical trials are classified as non-CTIMPs; for example, observational studies involving interviews or surveys. Whilst there is no legislation advising that non-CTIMPs should be conducted in accordance with GCP, it is always important to conduct research with the same principles in mind, in order to produce high-quality data and to protect the safety of the subjects enrolled in the trial. This is outlined in an additional framework; the UK Policy Framework for Health and Social Care Research (2017). This framework

requires all research to be performed to a high standard, regardless of the focus or methodology.

4.4.2 **Study personnel and roles**

When planning and conducting a research study, it is important to consider the different team members involved and their roles and responsibilities. These are summarised in *Table 4.2*.

Table 4.2: **A summary of study personnel, roles and responsibilities**

	Individual or organisation	Roles and responsibilities
Study sponsor	An organisation or partnership Commonly NHS Foundation Trusts or Universities	1. Responsible for the initiation, management and financing of the clinical study 2. Ensuring that insurances, indemnities, registrations and approvals are in place 3. Ensuring that research is carried out to a high standard and in accordance with GCP
Chief investigator (CI)	An individual who takes the overall lead for the research project	1. Takes primary responsibility for ensuring the conduct of the trial 2. Can delegate certain tasks and duties, but always remains responsible for them
Principal investigator (PI)	An individual who takes responsibility for the conduct of research at a study site In single-site studies, the PI and the CI are normally the same person	1. Responsible for the initiation and conduct at the study site 2. Responsible for participant recruitment, resource management, completion and management of delegation logs and the maintenance of adequate and accurate source documents
Site team	A range of individuals, e.g. clinical staff, pharmacists and lab workers	1. Everyone in the site team has a responsibility to ensure the safety and wellbeing of the study participants 2. Team members must comply with the research protocol, fulfil assigned duties and raise any issues to the PI

Throughout your medical career, it is possible to take different roles within a research study. As a junior doctor, you may form part of the site team and be delegated to recruit study participants or to complete study visits. If you undertake a career in academia, you may progress to become a PI or CI. Most of the positions are filled by consultant physicians.

4.4.3 Research approvals

Prior to a research study commencing, two main types of approval need to be obtained: ethical approval and sponsor approval.

Ethical approval is needed prior to starting a research study. This contrasts to projects involving service evaluation or audit, where this is not needed. In some cases, you may be uncertain whether your project falls into the remit of research or audit, and the Health Research Authority (HRA) has published an online decision tool which determines whether a study is classified as research or audit. When the study is classified as research, ethical approval is essential. The HRA tool outlines exactly what approvals are needed and whether submission to an NHS research ethics committee (REC) is required. When REC approval is needed, a study protocol and study documents are submitted electronically through the Integrated Research Application System (IRAS). If the protocol or study documents change during the course of the trial, they need to be resubmitted to the REC. This is discussed in more detail in *Section 4.11*.

In some studies, additional ethical approvals are needed. Most notably, CTIMPs require MHRA approval. During your medical career, it is important to work alongside your local research office to prepare applications for MHRA approval. Additional approvals are needed when research involves ionising radiation, new medical devices or human embryos.

Sponsor approval takes place after ethical approval is granted. In order for this to occur, the sponsor receives a copy of the REC's opinion. This dictates which protocol and study documents can be used in the trial.

4.5 Governance and ethical considerations during the study

During the course of the research study, there are many governance and ethical considerations to consider. We will discuss these throughout the next part of the chapter.

4.5.1 Subject recruitment and informed consent

Informed consent is of utmost importance in clinical research and is vital to ensure that the rights of subjects are protected. Legally, informed consent is necessary for valid insurance/indemnity. Without informed consent, participants and/or family can take legal action.

Informed consent is a two-step process that involves the following:

Step 1: Giving information

The individual must be given the information outlining their potential involvement in the clinical trial. In most cases, information is given verbally in the first instance and patients are subsequently given written information that takes the form of the **patient information leaflet (PIL)**. Once the individual has been given the information, they are under no pressure to respond and should be given time to consider their involvement in the trial.

Step 2: Gaining consent

After the individual has had a reasonable amount of time to consider their involvement in the trial, usually at least 24 hours, consent can be obtained by the researcher. In clinical research, written consent is required before the enrolment into a trial. In order to achieve this, the researcher reiterates the terms involved and asks the individual to consent to each term prior to consenting to participate in the research study as a whole. This is performed by means of a dated and signed informed consent form (ICF).

Important factors to consider during the consent process include the following:

- Consent must be voluntary, without coercion.
- Participants must be given sufficient time to consider their involvement in a clinical trial and have the opportunity to ask questions about their recruitment.
- Consent is ongoing throughout the research study and subjects have the right to withdraw informed consent at any point and for any reason.
- In order for valid consent to be obtained, individuals must have capacity to understand, retain and weigh their involvement in the clinical study.
- Alternatives to written consent forms can be considered. eConsent is a newer method of consent where participants can provide informed consent via an electronic signature, given through a tablet or other electronic device. In some cases, this can replace the traditional paper form.

4.5.2 Gaining consent in special cases

Sometimes it is not possible to obtain informed consent from study participants. This is often the case in studies involving children or vulnerable adults, such as adults with learning difficulties or dementia. When patients cannot give informed consent, consent is obtained from a third party, either the parent of a child or a consultee for a vulnerable adult. There are additional ethical complexities to be considered when recruiting children and vulnerable adults to clinical trials. The GCP outlines comprehensive guidelines in this area (NIHR Learn: https://learn.nihr.ac.uk).

WORKED EXAMPLE
A practical guide to designing PILs and consent forms

In order to obtain ethical approval, it is important to design a well-structured patient information leaflet (PIL) and consent form. The following worked example illustrates the important features and considerations when creating these forms. These forms were used in a study comparing the immune response against SARS-CoV-2 in individuals with autoimmune disease to those without. The following forms were sent to healthy individuals who had previously been infected with SARS-CoV-2.

Patient Information Leaflet (PIL)

Study Title:

Chief Investigator: REC ref:

Introduction
You are being invited to participate in a research study. Before you decide whether to take part, it is important to understand why the research is being done and what it will involve for you.

Please read the following information carefully and discuss it with others if you wish. We will go through the information sheet with you and answer any questions you have. We would suggest this would take about 20 minutes.

- Part 1 tells you the purpose of this study and what will happen to you if you take part.

- Part 2 gives you more detailed information about the conduct of the study.

Please ask if there is anything that is not clear. Take time to decide whether or not you wish to take part.

The PIL should be written on headed paper including the name of the organisation which is sponsoring the study.

The PIL should be titled with the study name, the name of the chief investigator and the REC reference.

A brief introduction outlines the purpose of the PIL and invites the reader to ask questions if anything is uncertain.

The purpose of the study should be explained to the patient. This should be written in layman's language.

The PIL outlines the reason why the patient has been invited to participate in the study.

The PIL emphasises that it is the participant's choice whether they take part in the study or not. The participant is informed that they can withdraw at any point and that participation will not affect their clinical care.

The PIL must explain exactly what the study involves for the patient.

Each page of the PIL should be labelled clearly with the title of the study, the version of the PIL and the date. This is usually included in the footer of the PIL alongside the page number and the IRAS ID.

PART 1
What is the purpose of the study?

With the recent coronavirus epidemic which has affected many parts of the world, people with arthritis, autoimmune conditions and inflammatory bowel disease who are on treatments with drugs that dampen down the immune system have been concerned about whether it is acceptable to continue their treatments or not. In some studies, treatments such as hydroxychloroquine, tumour necrosis factor alpha, or TNF inhibitors, biologic drugs to interleukin-6 (IL-6) and janus kinase inhibitor drugs such as baricitinib and tofacitinib are being proposed as treatments for coronavirus. In this study we want to find out if individual people with arthritis or inflammatory bowel disease have had symptoms of coronavirus and if we can detect signs of the virus infection from blood tests when people are on the type of treatments summarised above.

The Doctor will ask you questions about symptoms of Covid-19 and whether you have had the infection. If you are suitable for the study, you will be invited to participate. The study will involve answering questions that the Doctor or Nurse will ask you and giving blood to have a blood test. The blood test will measure antibodies to Covid-19 to see if you have had the infection.

Why have I been invited?

You have been invited to participate in this study as a healthy volunteer. We intend to compare your symptoms of Covid-19 and your antibody levels to patients with autoimmune disease.

Do I have to take part?

No. It is up to you to decide whether or not to take part. We will describe this study and go through this information sheet. If you do decide to participate, you will be given this information sheet to keep and asked to sign a consent form. You are still free to withdraw at any time and without giving a reason. A decision to withdraw at any time or not to take part will not affect the standard of care you receive. Participation in this study will also not alter your normal clinical care.

What will happen to me if I take part?
Prior to the study

If you choose to participate, one of the researchers carrying out the study will ask you to sign a consent form which will allow us to consider you for the study.

During the study

For the study, you will need to attend 2 appointments. The Doctor or Nurse who is seeing you will ask you some questions so they can complete a questionnaire about your symptoms. After completing the questionnaire, you will be asked to have a blood test. During the second visit, the Doctor or Nurse will take a second blood test. Both blood tests will measure the immune response to Covid-19 infection. The results of the blood tests will be compared to see if there is any change with time.

[Footer: Study Title, Version number and date, Page Number, IRAS ID]

What are the disadvantages and risks of taking part?

You will be having two blood tests, which are a couple of teaspoons of blood. The blood will be analysed to look for a response to infection to Covid-19 in your blood.

Blood test

The blood test may cause a little discomfort (a sharp scratch upon needle insertion) and some patients may experience a little bruising where the cannula (or small needle) is placed in the vein in the arm.

Study-related questionnaire

There is one questionnaire asking you about your condition, what your symptoms are, what treatment you are on and some more detailed questions about symptoms. This will take approximately 15 minutes, which you may find inconvenient.

What are the benefits of taking part?

This study aims to better understand how people who have arthritis, autoimmune conditions or inflammatory bowel disease may have had coronavirus, or not. We will gather this information from the questionnaire and blood tests. It will help us inform patients about infections such as coronavirus when they are on treatments that affect the immune system. The information we collect from this study may help us is providing future advice on their treatment for coronavirus.

What happens when the research study stops?

We plan to provide all the study participants with an update of the findings from our research at the end of the study. Participation in this study will not affect your routine clinical management.

Expenses and payments

We regret that we are not allowed to give you any financial incentive or payment for participation in our study. Information required for the study will be collected during your routine clinic visits so no additional travel expenses will be incurred.

What if there is a problem?

Any complaint about the way you have been dealt with or any possible harm you might suffer will be addressed. The detailed information on this is given in Part 2.

Will my taking part in the study be kept confidential?

Yes, we will follow ethical and legal practice and all information about you will be handled in confidence. The details are included in Part 2.

This completes Part 1

We hope that the information in Part 1 has interested you. If you are considering participation, please read the additional information in Part 2 before making your decision.

The risks of study participation must be explained. When blood is taken, it must be quantified using measurements such as "teaspoons of blood".

An explanation of what happens after the study is completed is provided.

It should be clearly explained whether expenses or payments are given to participating individuals. A decision on this must be made prior to starting the trial.

Participants are informed that the study results are kept confidential.

It is important to include a section in the PIL that outlines the procedure when participants no longer want to participate in the trial. This should include consideration as to the storage of samples that have already been collected.

The PIL must always contain a section explaining what to do if the participant wants to complain. In the first instance, the participant should be directed to the research team. In the case that this does not resolve the issue, the participant should be directed to the local PALS team.

The PIL outlines the procedure for compensation if injuries occur as a result of the trial.

It is important to explain how confidentiality is maintained and how personal information is kept safe.

PART 2

What will happen if I don't want to carry on with the study?

You can withdraw from the study at any time. You do not have to tell us the reason why; however, we would like to know for our records. Withdrawal from this study would not affect your usual treatment or care received here during or after the trial.

If you ask us to do so, we will destroy blood and urine samples collected so far. As we would prefer to keep the data and any samples collected already we would ask your permission to do so, but we would not collect any more.

What if I wish to complain about the trial?

If you wish to complain, or have any concerns about the way you have been treated during this study, then you can talk to the research team who will do their best to answer your questions or concerns. The National Health Service complaints mechanisms are also available to you.

The relevant NHS Patient Advice and Liaison Service (PALS) are on Tel.: [......]

What if there is a problem during or following my participation in the trial?

[...] NHS Trust / University has agreed that if you are harmed as a result of your participation in the study, you will be compensated, provided that, on the balance of probabilities, an injury was caused as a direct result of the intervention or procedures you received during the course of the study. These special compensation arrangements apply where an injury is caused to you that would not have occurred if you were not in the trial. We would not be bound to pay compensation where the injury resulted from a drug or procedure outside the trial protocol and/or the protocol was not followed. These arrangements do not affect your right to pursue a claim through legal action.

How will we use information about you?

We will need to use information from you and your medical records for this research project.

This information will include your NHS number. People will use this information to do the research or to check your records to make sure that the research is being done properly.

People who do not need to know who you are will not be able to see your name or contact details. Your data will have a code number instead.

We will keep all information about you safe and secure.

Once we have finished the study, we will keep some of the data so we can check the results. We will write our reports in a way that no one can work out that you took part in the study.

What are your choices about how your information is used?

- You can stop being part of the study at any time, without giving a reason, but we will keep information about you that we already have.

- If you choose to stop taking part in the study, we would like to continue collecting information about your health from your hospital. If you do not want this to happen, tell us and we will stop.

- We need to manage your records in specific ways for the research to be reliable. This means that we won't be able to let you see or change the data we hold about you.

- If you agree to take part in this study, you will have the option to take part in future research using your data saved from this study.

Where can you find out more about how your information is used?

You can find out more about how we use your information

- at www.hra.nhs.uk/information-about-patients/
- our leaflet available from www.hra.nhs.uk/patientdata-andresearch
- by asking one of the research team
- by sending an email to [......]
- by ringing us on [......]

Will my GP be informed?

We will not be informing your GP that you have taken part in this study. If any of the routine clinical investigations reveal any incidental findings your GP will be informed in accordance with standard practice.

Future research

Anonymised data may be transferred to non-commercial/commercial collaborators for use in this research or future research studies approved by a Research Ethics Committee.

What will happen to my samples?

Following completion of this study and with your permission, blood collected during this study may be stored for future ethically approved studies in research laboratories housed at [......]. You will be asked to sign a specific section of the consent form if you are happy for your samples to be used for analysis in future ethically approved studies. Your identity will not be revealed at any stage and any samples will be fully anonymised so you could not be traced.

If you do not provide your specific consent for your samples to be retained for future studies then the samples will be destroyed in accordance with standard laboratory procedures.

The PIL explains how participating individuals can make choices about data storage.

It is important to give participants a range of contact details and sources of information. This allows them to fully consider their involvement in the trial and allows them to ask any questions that may arise.

The PIL should state whether the participant's GP is informed of their enrolment. It is important to inform GPs in trials investigating new medications. In observational studies, it may not be necessary to inform the GP.

If relevant, it is important to inform the participant that samples may be used in future studies. Consent is needed for this.

Participants should be informed of the plan for data analysis and dissemination. They should be given the opportunity to request the results of the study.

What happens when the study is complete?
Once all of the trial data has been collected, the research team will analyse the data. We intend to publish the results in scientific journals to make the results of the trial available to a wider audience. If you would personally like to know the outcome of the study, please inform us and we would be happy to provide this information. You will not be identified in any reports or literature.

Who has reviewed the study?
All research in the NHS is looked at by an independent group of people, called a Research Ethics Committee (REC), to protect your interests. This study has been reviewed and given favourable opinion by NRES Committee Research Ethics Committee.

The PIL should signpost participants to resources for further information, such as the PALS team.

Further information
If you would like advice from someone else about whether to take part in this study, you can talk to your own GP or discuss it with friends or family. Alternatively, you can talk to the Patient Advice and Liaison Service (PALS) on [......].

You will be given a copy of this information sheet and a copy of the signed consent form to keep.

Thank you for considering taking part in this study.

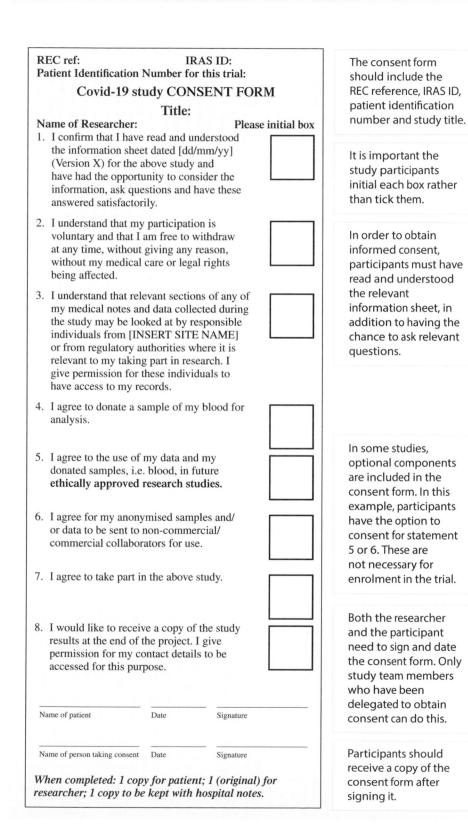

REC ref: IRAS ID:
Patient Identification Number for this trial:

Covid-19 study CONSENT FORM
Title:

Name of Researcher: Please initial box

1. I confirm that I have read and understood the information sheet dated [dd/mm/yy] (Version X) for the above study and have had the opportunity to consider the information, ask questions and have these answered satisfactorily.

2. I understand that my participation is voluntary and that I am free to withdraw at any time, without giving any reason, without my medical care or legal rights being affected.

3. I understand that relevant sections of any of my medical notes and data collected during the study may be looked at by responsible individuals from [INSERT SITE NAME] or from regulatory authorities where it is relevant to my taking part in research. I give permission for these individuals to have access to my records.

4. I agree to donate a sample of my blood for analysis.

5. I agree to the use of my data and my donated samples, i.e. blood, in future **ethically approved research studies.**

6. I agree for my anonymised samples and/or data to be sent to non-commercial/commercial collaborators for use.

7. I agree to take part in the above study.

8. I would like to receive a copy of the study results at the end of the project. I give permission for my contact details to be accessed for this purpose.

_____   _____   _____
Name of patient   Date   Signature

_____   _____   _____
Name of person taking consent   Date   Signature

When completed: 1 copy for patient; 1 (original) for researcher; 1 copy to be kept with hospital notes.

The consent form should include the REC reference, IRAS ID, patient identification number and study title.

It is important the study participants initial each box rather than tick them.

In order to obtain informed consent, participants must have read and understood the relevant information sheet, in addition to having the chance to ask relevant questions.

In some studies, optional components are included in the consent form. In this example, participants have the option to consent for statement 5 or 6. These are not necessary for enrolment in the trial.

Both the researcher and the participant need to sign and date the consent form. Only study team members who have been delegated to obtain consent can do this.

Participants should receive a copy of the consent form after signing it.

4.6 The use of placebo, blinding and randomisation to study arms

In RCTs, participants are randomised to control or intervention arms. In many cases, participants randomised to the control arm receive placebo. In RCT design, the ethical implications of placebo must be considered. When placebo is used, participants are deprived of active treatment and this has the potential of causing harm. When comparing placebo to active therapy, there are some trial designs that can be used. For example, a crossover trial allocates participants into two arms. After a predefined period of time, participants cross into the other arm, hence both groups receive active therapy for a certain time period. Another option is an 'add-on' design when both groups receive standard therapy, in addition to the experimental treatment or placebo.

4.6.1 The ethics of early study termination due to treatment benefit

In studies comparing two treatments, direct comparison is only ethical if it is unclear which treatment is more effective prior to the RCT taking place. This is called the principle of equipoise. In some cases, interim analysis demonstrates a significant benefit of one treatment over the other. In these cases, investigators feel obliged to stop the trial early to protect the interests of trial participants, some of whom are receiving an inferior treatment. Unfortunately, there are some downsides associated with this and it has been shown that studies that stop early, on average, overestimate treatment benefits due to a smaller number of accrued events. This highlights the ethical complexities involved in clinical research and the opposing requirements for scientific validity and social value versus protection of the study participants.

4.6.2 The ethics of blinding

Participants should only be unblinded for safety reasons, based on medical need. Except in emergency cases, this should be discussed with the sponsor. When a decision to unblind participants has occurred it should be documented clearly, including the reasons for unblinding.

WORKED EXAMPLE: early study termination due to treatment benefit
Dapagliflozin in patients with chronic kidney disease

Heerspink *et al.* (2020) *NEJM*, 383: 1436, doi.org/10.1056/NEJMoa2024816

Study aim

This study aimed to investigate the effects of dapagliflozin in patients with chronic kidney disease.

Methods

4304 participants with chronic kidney disease were randomised to receive 10mg daily dapagliflozin versus placebo. The primary outcome events included a decline in glomerular filtration rate (GFR) of at least 50%, the development of end-stage renal failure (ESRF) or death from renal or cardiovascular causes.

Results

The trial was terminated early due to the observed significant efficacy of dapagliflozin. At a median of 2.4 years post-enrolment, a primary outcome event had occurred in 197 of 2152 (9.2%) participants on dapagliflozin compared to 312 of 2152 (14.5%) participants on placebo. The number needed to treat to prevent the development of one primary adverse outcome was 19 (95% CI: 15 to 27). Participants allocated to receive dapagliflozin had significantly reduced risk of declining eGFR, ESRF or death. The benefit of dapagliflozin was similar in participants with and without type 2 diabetes.

Comments

- This trial was stopped early following a recommendation from an independent data monitoring committee. The committee deemed it unethical to continue to expose the subjects in the placebo arm to an inferior treatment. This may have reduced the power of some of the secondary outcomes.

4.7   Safety reporting

When conducting a clinical research trial, all staff should be familiar with the principles of safety reporting. It is vital that this information is collected in order to investigate the association between the study process, intervention or medication with any adverse events (AEs). By reporting AEs, we are protecting the safety of participants in the trial. For example, if patterns emerge to suggest that the intervention of interest is associated with a significant number of serious AEs, the trial may be terminated early.

After a participant has been enrolled in a research study, it is important to collect and record all AEs. This is the case regardless of whether or not the event is related to participation in the study. For example, imagine that during the study period, a participant falls and breaks their hip. Although this does not appear to be related to participation in the study, it is important to record nonetheless. This is the case with all unexpected AEs. In some cases, the recording of seemingly unrelated AEs in multiple participants will occur and raise the possibility that these are related in some way to participation in the trial.

CTIMPs are subject to additional safety reporting requirements. In these studies, serious adverse events (SAEs) require immediate reporting, within 24 hours of recording. Other AEs may require immediate reporting and if this is the case, this should be set out in the study protocol. Reporting of SAEs immediately is vital in order to ensure the safety of other participants enrolled in the study.

4.7.1 **Definitions of adverse events and severities**

Adverse event (AE): any unintended or untoward response in a study participant to whom an IMP has been administered. This includes events that are not necessarily related to that product and include symptoms, laboratory results and diseases. All AEs should be recorded in the source data (usually the medical notes) and in the **case report forms** (CRFs) or AE logs.

Adverse reaction (AR): any unintended or untoward reaction in study participants to IMPs or interventions. ARs differ from AEs in that there is at least a reasonable possibility that the reaction is due to the IMP.

Adverse events of special interest (AESI): AESIs are defined in the study protocol and include any noteworthy reaction for the particular drug or product under investigation.

Serious adverse event (SAE): SAEs are significant AEs that:

- result in death
- are life-threatening
- require inpatient hospitalisation
- result in significant disability
- result in congenital abnormalities or birth defects.

Suspected unexpected serious adverse reaction (SUSAR): this term relates to ARs reported in CTIMPs only. SUSARs describe ARs that are not consistent with the information known about the IMP; this is set out in the Reference Safety Information (RSI). Like SAEs and SARs, SUSARs must be reported to the sponsor immediately.

4.7.2 **Safety reporting and documentation**

All study personnel should know how to document AEs and this should be clearly set out in the study protocol. When reporting adverse events, it is important to document:

- The seriousness of the AE
  - i.e. whether the AE was serious or not
- The severity of the AE
  - this describes the intensity of the event and is usually classified as mild, moderate or severe
  - assessment of severity should be performed by a medically qualified person
- The causality of the AE
  - how likely is it that the event was related to the IMP? ARs differ from AEs in that there is at least a reasonable possibility that the reaction is due to the IMP
  - determining the causality of the AE requires medical and scientific judgement
- The expectedness of the AE
  - this is generally performed by the sponsor
  - this must be performed solely on the basis of the content of the approved RSI.

WORKED EXAMPLE: early study termination due to treatment harm
Maternal toxicity with continuous nevirapine in pregnancy

Hitti *et al.* (2004) *J Acquir Immune Defic Syndr*, **36**: 772, doi.org/10.1097/00126334-200407010-00002

Background

This study compared the safety of nelfinavir and nevirapine-based antiretroviral therapies in HIV-positive pregnant women.

Methods

In this study, 38 HIV-positive pregnant women were randomised to receive nelfinavir or nevirapine. These medications were given in combination with zidovudine plus lamivudine.

During the course of the study, it was noted that patients allocated to receive nevirapine developed greater than expected hepatic toxicity. Furthermore, new nevirapine prescribing information was released that recommended caution for women with CD4 counts greater than 250 cells per microlitre. This led the authors to perform an unscheduled interim analysis comparing treatment toxicity by arm, for all subjects and for the subgroup with a CD4 count greater than 250 cells per microlitre.

> **Comments**
>
> • By meticulously recording adverse events, study investigators noticed that participants enrolled to receive nevirapine experienced large numbers of adverse events. These events, in combination with the new prescribing information, led the study group to perform an interim analysis.

Results

Twenty-one subjects were randomised to receive nelfinavir and 17 subjects received nevirapine. Treatment-limiting toxicity (toxicity leading to the discontinuation of the study drug) was seen in 5% (1 of 21) on nelfinavir and 29% (5 of 17) subjects on nevirapine. Adverse events in the nevirapine group included one subject with Stevens–Johnson syndrome, two subjects with clinical hepatitis, one subject with asymptomatic raised ALT and one subject with fulminant liver failure and death. The liver biopsy results from the subject who died from fulminant liver failure were consistent with drug-induced hepatic toxicity. All of the subjects who developed toxicity had a CD4 count greater than 250 cells per microlitre. In all cases of hepatic toxicity, symptoms started 4–5 weeks after commencing nevirapine.

Discussion

This study was terminated early due to an increased rate of adverse events in patients receiving nevirapine. This study was limited by its small sample size; however, the toxicities observed were corroborated by previous case reports. Overall, this data raised serious concerns regarding the use of nevirapine in pregnant women with CD4 counts greater than 250 cells per microlitre.

> **Comments**
>
> • It would have been unethical to continue this study after the results from the interim analysis were released. In this case, the risk to study participants outweighed the benefit of study enrolment due to the unexpected severe adverse outcome (in this case hepatic toxicity).

4.8   Integrity throughout the study

Ethical and informative research requires high standards of integrity. Integrity requires the following:

- **Honesty** in all aspects of research, including data collection, data interpretation and data reporting
- **Excellence in research practice**, including the use of appropriate research methodology, adhering to relevant research protocols and analysing data in an appropriate manner.
- **Study transparency**, including the declaration of conflicts of interest, the transparent reporting of data collection and results and ensuring that results are widely available.
- **Adherence to the appropriate ethical, legal and professional frameworks.**

4.8.1 Examples of study misconduct

The World Association of Medical Editors (WAME) outlines seven categories of study misconduct:

1. *Falsification of data*, i.e. data fabrication, the omission of conflicting data and distortion of data.

2. *Plagiarism*, i.e. using ideas or language of others, without stating their true source.

3. *Inaccuracies in authorship*; for example, inclusion of authors who have not made definitive contribution to the work or the improper assignment of author contributions.

4. *Misappropriation of the ideas of others*.

5. *Violation of generally accepted research practices*; this includes deviations from accepted experimentation practices, deceptive statistical manipulations and deceiving reporting of results.

6. *Failure to comply with legal or regulatory requirements*.

7. *Inappropriate behaviour relating to misconduct*; this includes failure to report suspected misconduct or the destruction of information relevant to a claim of misconduct.

Other examples of study misconduct include:

- failure to declare conflicts of interest, e.g. funding or sponsorships
- duplicate publications
- failures of transparency.

4.9 Documentation, confidentiality and data protection

4.9.1 Study documentation

The GCP guidelines set out the criteria for accurate recording of source data and documentation. Specifically, data should be recorded to the standards of **ALCOAC**:

- **Attributable:** it should be clear who created the source record and when
- **Legible:** easy to read
- **Contemporaneous:** data should be recorded at the time that it is collected
- **Original:** i.e. the first documentation of the data or results; researchers are discouraged from transcribing or replicating source records
- **Accurate:** source records should be correct and valid
- **Complete:** there should be no omissions or censoring of data.

4.9.2 The investigator site file

The investigator site file (ISF) contains all of the documentation relating to the research study. *Table 4.3* outlines some of the key documents that are included within the ISF. It is the duty of the PI or a delegated team member to ensure that all documents are properly collated and updated throughout the study.

Table 4.3: A summary of the key documents included in the investigator site file

Document	Content
Study protocol/ amendments	The current protocol along with any historic protocols and protocol amendments should be included in the ISF
Standard operating procedure (SOP)	SOPs for experimental procedures
Patient information leaflet (PIL)	Current and historic PILs
Informed consent form (ICF)	Completed and signed ICFs
GP letters	Letters to GP to inform them of the subject's participation in trial
Letters of approval relating to site team	Documentation relating to ethical and sponsor approval
Training records and CVs of study team members	Generally speaking, all team members should have up-to-date GCP training with certificates included in the site file
	CVs from individuals listed on the delegation log should be included in the ISF
Delegation log	This summarises the individual members of the site team and which members are delegated to perform different tasks
	Start and end dates should be documented for all staff members
	All site team members should sign the delegation log

Case report form (CRF)	The CRF is a paper form, usually in the format of a questionnaire, to collect information from each participant
	The CRF should be complete, up-to-date and signed
Adverse events log	An up-to-date log of all AEs including the severity, expectedness and causality

4.9.3 Data protection

It is of utmost importance that the ISF is kept safely and securely. Data should be collected and recorded in accordance with the General Data Protection Regulation (GDPR) and Data Protection Act (2018). These are legal documents that dictate the reasons for data collection and how data can be stored. In order to collect personal data, organisations must have a valid and legal reason to process personal data. For health research, the basis is "task in public interest". When recording personal information, data must be anonymised or de-identified. This is most commonly done by replacing a person's name with a number.

4.10 Sampling and ethical considerations

In some clinical trials, human tissue is collected. The collection, storage and disposal of human tissue is governed by the Human Tissue Act (2004). This Act defined human tissue as any sample removed from a human body containing human cells. All staff working with human tissue must be aware of the relevant legislation. More information can be found at www.hta.gov.uk/guidance-professionals/hta-legislation/human-tissue-act-2004.

WORKED EXAMPLE
The UK Biobank

The UK Biobank is a large-scale database that stores in-depth genetic material and health-related information from half a million UK participants. Since 2006, the UK Biobank collected biological and medical data from individuals aged between 40 and 69 years old as part of a prospective study. All participating individuals provided consent for regular blood, urine and saliva samples, in addition to access to health-related records. Data from the biobank is anonymised and made accessible to researchers around the world, allowing them to perform studies on a range of different conditions.

While the UK Biobank has provided major contributions to the advancement of modern medicine, biobanking provides novel ethical considerations. Gaining informed consent is particularly difficult in studies using biobanking. This is because consent is taken as a 'one-off' process and does not address the long-term nature of biobanking. Furthermore, consent is not truly 'informed' as neither the participant nor researcher knows what research will be undertaken with the samples in the future.

4.11   Amendments

Changes in the study protocol after review body approval has been given are called amendments. Amendments can either be substantial or non-substantial. Different types of amendments require different approvals; this should be discussed with the PI or study coordinator. Amendments may need MHRA or REC approval. All amendments need to be tracked carefully. Examples of substantial amendments include:

- additional investigations or tests
- change in PI
- closure of a randomisation arm, e.g. if early data showed a significantly lower efficacy in one arm
- changes to the protocol or patient-facing documents (e.g. consent form or PIL).

4.12   Ethical considerations after the study

After the study is completed, it is vital that the results are reported accurately and ethically. When study results are reported poorly, data may be difficult to interpret. This can result in research waste and unnecessary duplication of trials.

4.13   Chapter summary

This chapter has highlighted the importance of planning and designing research studies and the documentation process that is involved in preparing necessary documents and approvals before research studies can be initiated. High-quality reporting is vital to ensure useful appraisal, evaluation and replication of study findings. This is needed to guide evidence-based clinical decision-making and policy-making.

4.14   Further reading

Declaration of Helsinki (1964): https://jamanetwork.com/journals/jama/fullarticle/1760318

HRA decision tool: www.hra-decisiontools.org.uk/research/

ICH Guidance for Good Clinical Practice E6 (R2) (2017): www.ema.europa.eu/en/ich-e6-r2-good-clinical-practice

NIHR Learn: https://learn.nihr.ac.uk (you will need a login to access this website)

Nuremberg Code: https://media.tghn.org/medialibrary/2011/04/BMJ_No_7070_Volume_313_The_Nuremberg_Code.pdf

UK Policy Framework for Health and Social Care Research (2017): www.hra.nhs.uk/planning-and-improving-research/policies-standards-legislation/uk-policy-framework-health-social-care-research/uk-policy-framework-health-and-social-care-research/

CHAPTER 5

Public and patient involvement

5.1   Introduction

5.1.1 What is public and patient involvement?

Public and patient involvement (PPI) is researchers working in active partnership with patients and the public to carry out research. This means carrying out research 'with' members of the public instead of 'to' them or 'for' them.

This is distinct from:

- **Participation:** the public/patients taking part in a research study.
- **Patient and public engagement (PPE):** disseminating research and creating a dialogue with the public/patients. Examples of PPE include science festivals open to the public with debates, research presentations open to the public, and raising awareness of research through social media and press.

Language

The language we use to describe PPI is different to language used to describe research. For example, terms such as 'interviewed' should not be used when describing consultations with the public, as this suggests a qualitative research study. This is a common mistake in many research grant applications describing PPI work. It is also important to ask the members of the public who are participating how they would like to be referred to. Terms such as 'participants' must not be used as these describe people taking part in a research study. Commonly used terms include 'PPI contributor' or 'PPI representative'.

5.1.2   Why is public and patient involvement important?

Patients are the most familiar with their condition as they have lived experience and can therefore provide unique and valuable insights which healthcare professionals and researchers may not be aware of. Therefore, involving patients ensures that the outcome of the research truly benefits patients.

Benefits to patient / the public

- Informs patients about research and enables them to feel more empowered that progress is being made in treating their condition

- Embodies principles of citizenship: as patients and the public are directly affected by health research, and contribute towards taxes which help to fund research, they have a right to know about it and have a say in how it is conducted
- Patients may want to 'give something back' after receiving publicly funded healthcare
- Can give a voice to seldom-heard groups
- Provides something interesting and challenging to take part in.

Benefits to researcher

- Can help with study recruitment and retention, because logistical issues and concerns that could affect potential participants will have already been discussed and resolved
- Improves the relevance and quality of research and ensures that it is most likely to have a real impact
- The importance of PPI is being increasingly recognised; this is reflected by many funding bodies now requiring evidence of PPI in funding applications.

5.2 How can the public and patients be involved in research?

5.2.1 Levels of public involvement

The different approaches to PPI based on Arnstein's Ladder of Citizen Participation are described below. As you travel down the ladder increasing levels of public involvement are described. A research project may involve a combination of these approaches.

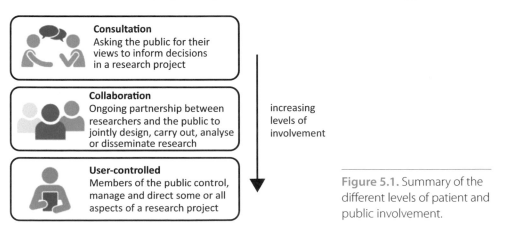

Consultation
Asking the public for their views to inform decisions in a research project

Collaboration
Ongoing partnership between researchers and the public to jointly design, carry out, analyse or disseminate research

User-controlled
Members of the public control, manage and direct some or all aspects of a research project

increasing levels of involvement

Figure 5.1. Summary of the different levels of patient and public involvement.

Table 5.1 shows some real extracts from PPI sections of NIHR funding applications. These exemplify the various approaches of PPI as well as examples of descriptions which cannot be classed as PPI.

Table 5.1: Extracts from PPI sections of NIHR grant applications

Example	Consul-tation	Collab-oration	User-controlled	Not PPI	Comments
We plan a steering group for the project with four patient representatives as equal members of the research team		✓			
In the first phase of the study 10 [patients] and 5 carers will be invited to participate in semi-structured interviews. They will be asked their thoughts and perceptions of the [intervention]. Results from the first phase of the study will influence the second phase, a randomised controlled trial.				✓	'semi-structured interviews' describes a qualitative research method; 'participate' describes participation in research; 'results' describes study data. Therefore this is classified as a qualitative research.
A steering committee subgroup comprising solely users and carers supported by researchers will be asked to direct planning of methods and content whereby user and carer views of service delivery will be obtained and evaluated			✓		
Our patients agreed with us that the study would deliver important information and that the research was timely and important	✓				'agree with us' suggests poor PPI. Consultations should be used to gain patients' / the public's view and use them to shape research, instead of presenting pre-made plans.

Table provided courtesy of Dr Duncan Barron, St George's, University of London.

WORKED EXAMPLE: Consultation
A multi-centre programme of clinical and public health research to guide health service priorities for preventing suicide in England

Lead researcher: Professor David Gunnell, University of Bristol

www.invo.org.uk/wp-content/uploads/2013/10/Example-9-public-involvement-in-funding-application-2013.pdf

Background

This project aimed to inform the National Suicide Prevention Strategy. A one-day workshop was held with potential end users including service users, representatives from the Samaritans, policy makers and NHS clinicians and managers to discuss research priorities for a grant proposal.

> ### Comment
> - The service users were involved in a previous grant as co-investigators and service users were reimbursed for their time with funds from the first grant.

The workshop shaped the grant proposal by the following actions:

- Increasing PPI in the project by involving more service user advisers, and broadening their role to include providing feedback on interview topic guides and question wording in pilot interviews.
- Developing clear policies around supporting service users involved in research due to the potential for this research topic to cause distress, such as ensuring lethal methods of suicide are not discussed around potentially vulnerable people.

> ### Comment
> - Involvement of service users in consultations can ensure that research is designed sensitively to minimise distress and maximise benefit to patients.

> *"One of the things the researchers wanted to look at was self-harm services. I suggested that they needed to include users of those services in that process so not just to look at hard outcomes, but also, for example, how relationships between users and staff influence the quality of care."* **Rosie Davies** [service user co-applicant on the Programme Grant]

WORKED EXAMPLE: Collaboration
Co-designing an intervention to strengthen vaccine uptake in Congolese migrants in the UK

Researchers: Alison Crawshaw (St George's, University of London) Caroline Hickey (Hackney Council for Voluntary Service), Hackney Congolese Women Support Group

Background

This study used community-based participatory research with Congolese migrants to co-design interventions to address barriers to vaccine uptake in this community. This involved forming a community–academic partnership to lead the study and the use of in-depth interviews, interactive posters, and community days with Congolese migrants to understand their experiences and beliefs on vaccination, as well as interviews with local clinical, public health and community stakeholders. The findings were discussed and interpreted in co-design workshops with the community to design interventions which were then delivered by the community.

> **Comment**
> * A co-design approach was chosen, as a tailored intervention was likely to be more effective due to this group having lower engagement with services and low trust in institutions.

How the study was conducted

1. The study began by conducting pre-engagement workshops in January/February 2021 with multiple community leaders from migrant and Black communities in Hackney to decide on a research problem related to vaccination that was identified by the community. The Congolese migrant community was identified as the target population for the study and preliminary insights about community perceptions about vaccines were gained. Contributors were financially compensated and recognised for their expertise / lived experience.

> **Comment**
> * These workshops invited members of migrant communities to contribute ideas of importance to their personal and community needs. Trust between the researchers and community was also built over a period of months.

2. A coalition of academic and community partners was formed to lead the study in November 2021. The group met for a total of approximately 20 hours to discuss expectations, roles and responsibilities, decide on the research question and approach, seek ethics approval, develop data collection tools and carry out pilot testing. Community members were trained as peer qualitative researchers, and study partners were financially compensated for their time and effort.

> **Comment**
> * Co-researcher training enabled contributors to effectively carry out their roles as well as addressing power imbalances between researchers and contributors. This is discussed more in *Section 5.3.2.*

3. Data collection occurred through 32 semi-structured interviews with Congolese migrants during three 'Community Days' to investigate beliefs and experiences in relation to catch-up and Covid-19 vaccinations. These were held in private rooms at a local community centre, which is near a local market that the Congolese community attends for shopping. These events included a social area with local cuisine, music and linkage to other community services and development opportunities. Interviews were conducted in local language (predominantly Lingala or French).

"They were welcoming and showing us what the project is about and also recognising and using the Congolese language" Participant from Congolese community

Comment
- The choice of peer-led data collection during community days fostered trust and enabled high engagement from the community. The learning and development opportunities offered upskilled and empowered community members to conduct future research of their own.

4. Seven In-depth online interviews with local stakeholders were held to understand local pathways and discuss possible interventions.
5. Co-analysis was conducted and Consensus workshops were held to discuss results. This led to a co-design workshop framework.
6. Two co-design workshops were conducted with 16 migrants where interventions and recommendations were defined.

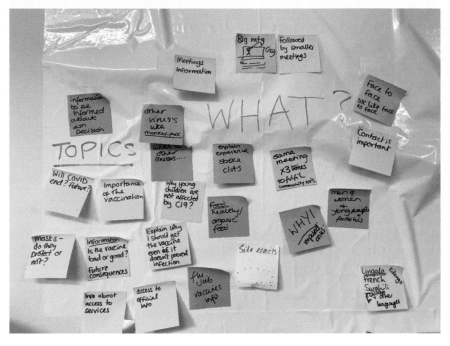

Figure 5.2. Feedback from the community during co-design workshops on what topics the intervention should include. Image reproduced with permission of Alison Crawshaw.

Three interventions were co-designed: short plays, community-led health dialogues / workshops, and posters to myth-bust and answer questions that were raised by the community about vaccination, all in local language.

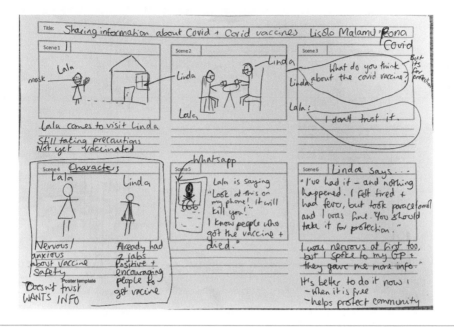

Figure 5.3. Storyboard planning the short play intervention co-designed by the Congolese community to encourage vaccine uptake. Image reproduced with permission of Alison Crawshaw.

Comment

- These interventions are more likely to be effective due to answering specific questions/concerns in a non-judgemental environment and being in a format that the community reported to be most engaging to them.

7. Dissemination of these interventions was conducted during a community celebration event where community members were invited to wear national dress and celebrate with food and music. This was attended by approximately 45 community members and a local councillor.

Comments

- These events help continue the partnerships for future research and maintain trust.
- This study demonstrates best practice in collaborative PPI by ensuring power sharing, employing financial compensation, recognition of lived experience and expertise, and upskilling the community. Research activities were met with positive feedback as contributors reported feeling valued and welcomed. This is an effective approach for dealing with the complex issue of low vaccine uptake in certain communities.

WORKED EXAMPLE: User-controlled
User-led research group: Wales mental health service

Lead researcher: Anne Fothergill, University of Glamorgan

A potential model for the first all Wales mental health service user and carer-led research group

Wilson *et al.* (2010) *J Psych Mental Health Nursing*, 17: 31, doi.org/10.1111/j.1365-2850.2009.01473.x

This example summarises how a service user and carer-led mental health research group was set up in Wales in 2008. This was the first group of this type in Wales.

How the user group was set up

1. Mental health service users and carers were invited to attend a one-day workshop called 'Getting Involved in Research' at the University of South Wales to explore their opinions on service user involvement. During the workshop, service users reported that they wanted to be involved in the local dissemination of research findings and one of the workshop delegates was invited to write a lay report about the workshop findings. It subsequently became obvious that the service user would require research and empowerment training in order to complete this task. After the report was published, the local borough council requested further training should be provided by the university.

2. Ten mental health service users with a range of illness severities took part in eight weekly research and empowerment training sessions, lasting 3 hours each, with 4 hours of homework per session.

   • **Empowerment training:** this was in the form of creative autobiographical writing which included writing stories and poems.

   • **Research training:** service users were provided with INVOLVE Public Information Pack booklets explaining involvement in research and research terminology.

3. After completion of the training courses, service users wrote down goals for future research objectives. Some examples included: developing models of wellness instead of illness, working with the local media to challenge mental health stigma, research into how general practitioners comply with NICE guidance and barriers to adhering to this.

> Comment
> • These training sessions boosted the confidence of the service users and equipped them with vital skills for carrying out research and expressing their views effectively. This example lays out a model of how to facilitate the formation of a user group through empowerment and research training.

Service user: *"The training really built up our confidence in many different aspects of our lives. We started off thinking of ourselves as 'service users', and then as 'consumers of services' and finally, towards the end of the training, we realized that we are 'expert patients' and 'expert citizens'. It really did help us to see that we have unique skills and abilities, and that we have something of value to give to society."*

Service user (Tina) *"The atmosphere quickly became very relaxed and enjoyable – after just two weeks. When we did some research training it was all very exciting. We were also given the opportunity of attending a conference in Bridgend where we helped to run a workshop for researchers to help them understand how to empower people in research…. In the workshop we learned more about what it was like to be a 'researcher' and researchers were able to learn more about us – as patients and carers. It was an exciting way of helping us to break down barriers – everyone learned a lot and we enjoyed ourselves very much."*

5.2.2 Involvement throughout the research cycle

Patients and the public can be involved in all stages of a research project including the following.

Identifying and prioritising

- Holding a consultation with patients to identify research priorities or reaffirm the importance of previously identified research aims
- Asking organisations that support the public about the feedback they get from service users.

Identifying research priorities: James Lind Alliance (JLA) and priority setting partnerships (PSP)

The JLA facilitates priority setting partnerships (PSPs), which enable clinicians, patients and carers to identify and prioritise evidence uncertainties (questions which cannot be answered by existing research) collaboratively. They provide useful templates and documents to guide the formation of a PSP and can allocate a JLA adviser to help an organisation form a PSP.

Commissioning research

- Contributors reviewing research proposals
- Working with contributors on commissioning panels
- Contributors as co-applicants for a research proposal.

Example co-applicant on a research proposal: Decision-making about implantation of cardioverter defibrillators (ICDs) and deactivation during end of life care

www.invo.org.uk/wp-content/uploads/2013/10/Example-4-publicinvolvement-in-funding-app2013.pdf

The research team submitted two grants which focused on decisions involving implantation of ICDs. These were both rejected, with feedback that this was not an area of patient need. The final grant utilised PPI and included recommendations from an experienced carer. The feedback was that decisions around deactivation and the timing of discussing these decisions were more important for patients than implantation of ICDs. This shifted the focus of the study considerably and resulted in the final grant application being accepted. The carer became a co-applicant on the grant and contributed to drafting the application.

Comment
- Patient/carer involvement can help increase the likelihood of grants being accepted, due to shaping the research focus to make it relevant for patient needs.

Designing research
- Comments on possible ethical and safety issues from a patient perspective
- Assessing the tolerability, appropriateness and logistics of trial interventions; for instance, scheduling research blood tests at the same time as routine blood tests
- Contributors helping to write plain English summaries of protocols
- Contributors providing feedback on perceived process of consent in a trial
- Contributors helping to design patient information leaflets and consent forms.

Example commenting on study materials: Bone and joint study

Quote from healthtalk.org: https://healthtalk.org/patient-and-public-involvement-research/what-activities-and-tasks-are-involved

"So because my daughter had a bone infection I'm the person that's been co-opted onto the largest bone joint study that will run in this country… I've been involved right from the very inception of the bone and joint study. And was even able to impact the graphics that they use to invite people to join the bone and joint study. They wanted to use this skeleton, the shape of a skeleton of a baby and I felt that skeletons were quite scary and having been subjected to my own bereavement, in my past, and being worried that my child, that my child might die when she had a bone infection, found that that was an emotional image. So the image was changed to a different one that was more fun and that was more appropriate for children as opposed to it being bones because it was about bones."

Comment
- Feedback on or co-design of patient information leaflets can uncover perspectives that researchers may not be aware of and encourage more study recruitment.

Data collection

- Contributors collecting survey data
- Contributors conducting interviews / focus groups with research participants
- Contributors carrying out library-based research
- Participant recruitment.

Example helping with recruitment:
Breast cancer study

Quote from healthtalk.org:

https://healthtalk.org/patient-and-public-involvement-research/carolyn-

"A couple of us also were, one of my colleagues was videoed and I did an audio, a podcast, as a patient giving my perspective to help in the set-up in the recruitment, something that people could click on a website and hear other patients' perspective and why we thought this was an important area to research."

Comment
- Patient involvement with recruitment can inspire other patients to take part in research.

Managing research

- Contributors helping with governance and assessing safety data
- Becoming members of patient advisory or steering group.

Patient advisory group member:
Una Rennard, member of NIHR INVOLVE Advisory Group

Una Rennard helped to produce the UK standards of public involvement in 2019, building upon INVOLVE Values and Principles Framework. She is also part of the NIHR TCC where she helps to interview candidates in consideration for funding.

Comment
- The public members of advisory or steering groups ensure the patient perspective is considered.

Quote from healthtalk.org:

"As a public contributor I want to ensure proposed research is asking questions that are important to patients and is acceptable to potential participants." Una Rennard

Analysing research

- Contributors checking conclusions from a public perspective and highlighting findings that may be relevant to the public
- Contributors analysing interview/survey data with the support of researchers.

Example analysing data:
The views and experiences of service users regarding illicit drug use in secure settings

Source: www.invo.org.uk/wp-content/uploads/documents/MHRN_CaseStudiesAugust_2013.pdf

Service users were involved in conducting and analysing interviews with illicit drug users in medium secure units. They were able to provide additional information; for example, telling researchers about cultural influences on substance abuse, as well as explaining the rationale behind things being said or not being said, such as how the service users may judge the staff's competency and its effect on situations.

> **Comment**
> - Involving service users can bring another perspective to analysis based on personal experiences, which may aid interpretations.

Dissemination

- Contributors ensuring that findings are presented in a way that the public can understand
- Contributors writing articles for patient charities
- Contributors disseminating research to patient groups
- Co-authoring academic publications.

Example disseminating to the public:
Presenting at conferences

Quote from healthtalk.org: https://healthtalk.org/patient-and-public-involvement-research/types-of-involvement#51622

"One of my jobs before I retired was as a teacher trainer, postgraduate certificate in education. So my job was to not only set an example, but assess people on presenting information in a way which would engage the audience and would convey the meaning effectively and hopefully permanently; it would stick. So I went to the first of these conferences and – fairly critical of the presentation skills of some of the presenters [laughs]. So I said in my lack of wisdom, you know, 'I don't think that was done very well.' So of course next year they said, 'Well you can do it then.' [Laughs]. Fortunately it was only a short slot that I was given, but yeah you see presentation skills – if you're going to sell your research project to the general public, there's a way of addressing people at that level, which is nothing like symposia language and it's a different type of speaking."

> **Comment**
> - Contributors bring a lay perspective to help ensure that researchers are communicating in terms that the public can understand. They can also help to present findings to other members of the public in an engaging way.

5.3 How to carry out effective PPI

5.3.1 UK Standards for Public Involvement in Research

The UK Standards for Public Involvement in Research are a framework for conducting good PPI established in July 2016 by representatives from the NIHR, Chief Scientist Office (Scotland), Public Health Agency (Northern Ireland), and Health and Care Research Wales.

Read more about the standards through this link: https://sites.google.com/nihr.ac.uk/pi-standards/home

The standards are outlined below:

Inclusive opportunities: "Offer public involvement opportunities that are accessible and that reach people and groups according to research needs"

Working together: "Work together in a way that values all contributions, and that builds and sustains mutually respectful and productive relationships"

Support and learning: "Offer and promote support and learning opportunities that build confidence and skills for public involvement in research"

Communications: "Use plain language for well-timed and relevant communications, as part of involvement plans and activities"

Impact: "Seek improvement by identifying and sharing the difference that public involvement makes to research"

Governance: "Involve the public in research management, regulation, leadership and decision making".

5.3.2 Practical considerations

This section will give an outline of some of the practical aspects to consider when conducting PPI; these will incorporate the standards described in *Section 5.3.1*.

When to start

Starting PPI as early as possible is highly recommended, to ensure as many involvement opportunities as possible throughout a research project. It also enables strong relationships with PPI contributors to be built, which is necessary for fruitful involvement and allows continued involvement in future research projects.

Setting up involvement opportunities

Researchers should not have a formal recruitment process, as PPI emphasises that anyone can be involved; however, sometimes it may be important for the contributor to have certain experience and skills depending on the PPI role. Clearly outlining what the involvement will entail and why you require a patient perspective is useful and will nurture a productive partnership. This could involve creating a job description with responsibilities and time commitment expectations; it is important for clarify what is expected of PPI contributors.

It's important to involve people from a variety of demographics and backgrounds, including harder to reach people, to reflect the needs of the whole community. Therefore, careful consideration should be made regarding practical barriers inhibiting involvement, such as people with care or childcare responsibilities, travel costs for people with low income, and patients with chronic health conditions who find it hard to manage their responsibilities alongside their conditions. In order to be inclusive, researchers need to adapt the sessions to allow more flexible involvement and advertise in an accessible manner. Involvement opportunities which are visible and accountable should be offered throughout the organisation, and adequate resources (including staff time and funding) should be allocated before commencement.

Common methods of recruitment

- NHS clinics, GP surgeries
- Existing/previous participants from research studies
- Support groups, charities
- Social media (Instagram, Facebook, Twitter)
- Youth clubs and schools
- Personal contacts
- Groups and websites such as people in research, research design service, biomedical research centres, centre for public engagement, clinical research networks
- Asking PPI contributors to refer others.

Communications

When communicating with PPI contributors, it's vital that lay English is used and jargon is avoided. Ensure that a variety of communication mediums are used to maximise accessibility, e.g. offering posted information for those who do not have access to a computer or printer, as well as considering translating communications for those who do not speak English as a first language. Additionally, it is important to offer feedback opportunities for PPI contributors to share their thoughts about their experience of involvement. This feedback should then be shared and acted on to improve PPI practice.

Meetings

Good chairing during PPI meetings is necessary to ensure meetings are productive, welcoming and that everyone has an equal chance to speak. Circulation of meeting agendas and minutes ensures that everyone is well informed about what was covered and what needs to be done, and can help PPI contributors stay motivated due to their input being documented. Offering refreshments or catering at meetings also creates a welcoming environment.

Virtual PPI

Offering virtual PPI opportunities is important to provide flexible involvement opportunities for those with time constraints. Since the coronavirus pandemic, certain patient groups – such as cancer patients receiving immunosuppressive therapies – may feel vulnerable attending in-person sessions. Virtual sessions are more accessible for people who have concerns about paying for transport and may allow people with relevant experiences to come together and contribute, e.g. patients of a very rare disease could easily meet without travel time. Downsides of virtual PPI include reduced accessibility to people who are not confident using computers, people with no internet access and people who are not comfortable appearing in front of a camera. It may also feel less personal than in-person meetings.

Payment

It is important to reimburse PPI contributors for their time and effort; this is usually done through payment for their time and reimbursement for expenses such as travel, overnight accommodation, childcare costs, etc. The NIHR has guidance about the right level of payment for specific tasks such as reviewing research briefs, attending an advisory committee and attending meetings/teleconferences according to the time spent.

Ethical considerations

INVOLVE ethical statement: "You do not need to apply for ethical approval to involve the public in the planning or the design stage of research, for example helping to develop a protocol, questionnaire or information sheet, being a member of a research advisory group, or preparing an application for funding or ethical review, even when those people are approached for this role via the NHS".

This is because they are not acting as research participants, and you are not collecting data from them to be published.

Situations that may raise ethical concerns:
- The wellbeing of patients actively involved as researchers, since talking to people with their condition may remind them of negative personal experiences and cause distress. In this case additional support/counselling may be required.
- If involvement involves direct contact with participants in the study, the safety, wellbeing, and preferences of study participants must be considered. For example, they may prefer to be recruited by study staff as opposed to other patients. The patient / member of the public must also have adequate training, support and supervision.

Training

> **Put yourself in the public's shoes:** imagine entering an academic environment for the first time and being asked to work with professors, clinicians and statisticians. You may feel like you are not qualified to contribute to research due to your lack of scientific background. Additionally, hearing lots of unfamiliar terminology may feel intimidating.

The public's 'lay' view is an important aspect for PPI so on one hand, too much training may diminish this outsider perceptive. On the other hand, PPI activities can be daunting for the public, and asking them to undertake activities with no training is not reasonable. Training can also ensure an equal balance of power between researchers and contributors. As well as formal training sessions, there should be signposting to resources available for the public to seek information and support if necessary. Training and learning should be an ongoing process where advice is shared within the organisation, in order to learn from past experiences.

Training requirements for contributors

- Research terms and abbreviations
- Research ethics and Good Clinical Practice
- How to contribute effectively during meetings
- Time management
- Managing emotions
- Role-specific training.

Reporting on PPI

The Guidance for Reporting the Involvement of Patients and the Public (GRIPP) is an evidence-based international guidance tool for the reporting of PPI. This contains checklists of key items that researchers should include in publications to promote high quality, transparent and consistent reporting of PPI. A three-round Delphi survey was used to decide which items should be included and this led to the creation of short-form and long-form versions. The long-form version, GRIPP2-LF, contains 34 items on aims, definitions, concepts and theory, methods, stages and nature of involvement, context, capture or measurement of impact, outcomes, economic assessment and reflections.

5.4 Assessing the impact of PPI

5.4.1 Why assess impact?

It's crucial to measure the impact of PPI in order to improve the quality of PPI and provide evidence that the benefits outweigh the costs, to provide evidence for future funding. Evidence of impact can also aid research being taken up by policy makers and encourage more involvement from the public by proving that their involvement has made a difference.

Tokenistic PPI is when researchers carry out PPI as a 'tick box' exercise and undertake poor PPI that does not add value to a study in order to fulfil grant application requirements. This may be carried out by researchers who are sceptical about the value of PPI or feel that their professional status is being undermined by contributors. This can be a self-fulfilling prophecy. In order to reduce PPI scepticism, evidence of the positive impacts of PPI must be published.

5.4.2 Public Involvement Impact Assessment Framework

Due to the many approaches to PPI in a variety of contexts, assessing the impact of PPI can be difficult and a general approach cannot be used. The Public Involvement Impact Assessment Framework (PiiAF) sets out a method to assess the impact of PPI which involves firstly considering the influence of different factors on the impacts of the PPI (Part 1) then creating a specific assessment plan (Part 2). The example below shows how a research group implemented the PiiAF.

> **WORKED EXAMPLE:**
> **The Spectrum Centre for Mental Health Research**
>
> **Using the Public Involvement Impact Assessment Framework to assess the impact of public involvement in a mental health research context: a reflective case study**
>
> Collins *et al.* (2018), *Health Expectations*, 21: 950, doi.org/10.1111/hex.12688
>
> The Spectrum Centre for Mental Health Research was set up at Lancaster University in 2008 and focuses on developing psychological approaches to supporting people with severe mental health problems. A steering group was set up between January and September 2014 to assess the impact of service user involvement activities in the Spectrum Centre group and assess the use of the PiiAF.
>
> *PiiAF Part 1: aspects to consider when planning impact assessment*
>
> *In Part 1 researchers must consider aspects which may affect the impact of PPI, such as:*
> * *values held by researchers or organisations associated with PPI*
> * *approach to PPI*

- *research design and study population*
- *practical issues, including availability of training and resources, issues with payment for involvement.*

Part 1 ends with identifying feasible impacts of the involvement.

In order to carry out Part 1 of the PiiAF, the steering group administered an audit tool based on the PiiAF record card to identify the purpose, processes, impacts, context and assessment of PPI. This was emailed to staff members in the Spectrum Centre ($n = 15$) and all members of the Service User Advisory Panel ($n = 12$).

A summary of responses is shown below (reproduced under a Creative Commons CC BY licence):

Recording key points from your discussion

Values   Why do public involvement (PI)?

- To increase the relevance and improve the quality of research
- To ensure the language used is appropriate and understandable across a range of audiences
- To influence policy
- To ensure knowledge is shared/disseminated appropriately
- To give a voice to the 'public'

Approaches to PI Different ways that PI is undertaken currently
Involvement in:

- Staff training
- Study design
- Intervention development and design
- Research as participants
- Recruitment of research participants
- Dissemination of results (in a variety of ways)
- As grant holders / co-applicants

Practical issues What wider influences have shaped PI work at the Spectrum Centre?

- National bodies / research frameworks, e.g. INVOLVE
- Internet and social media
- Involvement of people with lived experience of bipolar disorder (service users, relatives and carers) in the Spectrum Centre

What practical issues have shaped PI work at the Spectrum Centre?

- Problems with financial support for service users involved in different ways
- Trying to establish appropriate structures to support, manage and organise PI: Advisory Panel and Spectrum Connect
- Important that people are paid for their involvement but should not undervalue the importance of voluntary involvement as well. Rules governing welfare payments may impose some limits on the amount of work people are able to do.

**Identifying the
impacts of PI in
research**

How does PI affect the research process and conclusions?

- Increases relevance
- Increases validity
- Increases credibility
- Reduces stigma

What difference does PI make?

- Foregrounds the lived experience of bipolar disorder
- Opens a wider audience for the research

How do you think PI could be assessed at the Spectrum Centre?

- Questionnaires and feedback
- Monitor PI

Following the audit tool, all staff members and service users on the Advisory Panel were invited to take part in a workshop to expand on their responses.

PiiAF Part 2: Developing an impact assessment plan

Part 2 is divided into the following stages:

1. **Foundations phase:** *decide on why you are carrying out the impact assessment, e.g. do you want to improve the PPI process? Do you want to identify factors affecting the PPI process? Do you want to demonstrate the outcomes of PPI?*
   In this stage you can decide if members of the public or research team will carry out the impact assessment.

> Comments
> - The team used a variety of tables provided in the PiiAF guidance document. The reasons for assessing impact were discussed in steering group meetings and it was agreed that all members of the Centre should have the opportunity to contribute.

2. **Developing your intervention theory:** *how could your PPI approach lead to the impacts you want? For example, how may your PPI approach increase recruitment onto a trial?*
3. **Identifying possible effects of context on impacts of public involvement:** *how do research design, values and practical issues affect these impacts? These can be positive or negative.*

Firstly, possible impacts were identified using a database search of similar studies:

- PPI impact on service user pathways for engagement with the Spectrum Centre
- PPI impact on research agenda setting
- PPI impact on the interpretation of findings
- PPI impact on the dissemination of findings.

Then the way in which PPI in the Spectrum Centre could lead to desired impacts was discussed; for example, to develop specific intervention theories and assessment plans; see *Table 5.2.*

Table 5.2: Intervention theory and impact assessment plan

Intervention theory	Impact assessment plan
PPI impact on research agenda setting: PPI through service user researchers (SURs) ensures that research priorities are more relevant as a result of research project proposals being informed by lived experience of people with bipolar disorder	Explore similarities and differences in research priorities between Spectrum Centre academics and SURs Use qualitative methods to explore perceptions of relevance

4. ***Formulating assessment questions and study design:*** *think about who, how and what.*

Table 5.3: Breaking down the assessment question into parts of who, how and what

WHO?	HOW?	WHAT?
Service users	Developing research priorities	Increase research relevancy

Final question: Does involving service users as SURs collaborating with academics on research priority development in the Spectrum Centre lead to proposals that are perceived by key stakeholder groups to be more relevant and informed by lived experience of bipolar disorder?

> **Comment**
> - Then researchers must decide on how impact will be measured, e.g. qualitative or quantitative methods, and what data collection method and indicators will be used.

Indicators and measures were developed (see *Table 5.4*).

Table 5.4: Summary of intervention theory and impact assessment plan, including indicators of impact and how the data will be collected

Intervention theory	Impact assessment plan	Impact assessment question	Identify indicators	Develop measures	Data
PI impact on research agenda setting: PI through service user researchers (SURs) ensures that research priorities are more relevant as a result of research project proposals being informed by lived experience of people with bipolar disorder	Explore similarities and differences in research priorities between Spectrum Centre academics and SURs. Use qualitative methods to explore perceptions of relevance	Does involving service users on research priority development in the Spectrum Centre lead to proposals that are perceived to be more relevant to key stakeholder groups?	Differences in research priorities proposed by SURs and academics	Ratings of relevance made by key stakeholder groups outside the research team, including service users and grant funders	Qualitative–thematic coding of identified priorities (e.g. Brown *et al.*, 2006) Ratings of relevance from key stakeholder groups

Comments
- This step-by-step example showed how researchers can apply the PiiAF to plan how the impact from PPI will be measured. The service users and researchers carrying out the impact assessment used a reflective framework to capture their experiences of using PiiAF and found the process useful overall. For more insight into some of the challenges they encountered, see www.ncbi.nlm.nih.gov/pmc/articles/PMC6250886.

5.5 Chapter summary

This chapter has described what is meant by patient and public involvement and how this is distinct from engagement activities and participatory research. It has described the practicalities of conducting involvement activities and emphasises the importance of thinking about this early in a research project to build strong relationships and encourage future involvement opportunities. Finally, it has outlined how to conduct effective patient and public involvement and how to measure its impact.

5.6 References and useful resources

Arnstein's Ladder of Citizen Participation: about citizen involvement in planning processes in the USA – *Journal of the American Planning Association*, 1969; 35: 216.

BMJ evaluating impact: www.bmj.com/content/363/bmj.k5147

Brown, K. *et al.* (2006) Discovering the research priorities of people with diabetes in a multicultural community: a focus group study. *BJGP*, **56(524):** 206–13.

Cambridge Biomedical Research Centre advisory groups: https://cambridgebrc.nihr.ac.uk/wp-content/uploads/2017/03/PPI-panel-focus-groups.pdf and https://cambridgebrc.nihr.ac.uk/public/the-cuh-ppi-panel/

healthtalk – examples of PPI from healthtalk: https://healthtalk.org/patient-and-public-involvement-research/what-activities-and-tasks-are-involved

Improving inclusion: www.nihr.ac.uk/documents/improving-inclusion-of-under-served-groups-in-clinical-research-guidance-from-include-project/25435

INVOLVE was a national advisory group funded by the NIHR that no longer exists; however, many of its resources are still available online. It has now been superseded by the NIHR Centre for Engagement and Dissemination: www.invo.org.uk/

INVOLVE ethical statement: www.invo.org.uk/wp-content/uploads/2016/05/HRA-INVOLVE-updated-statement-2016.pdf

INVOLVE guide to co-production: www.invo.org.uk/wp-content/uploads/2019/04/Copro_Guidance_Feb19.pdf

James Lind Alliance: www.jla.nihr.ac.uk/

NHS info on PPI: www.england.nhs.uk/aac/what-we-do/patient-and-public-involvement/

NIHR guidance for organisations on determining the most appropriate payment approach: www.nihr.ac.uk/documents/Payment-for-Public-Involvement-in-Health-and-Care-Research-A-guide-for-organisations-on-determining-the-most-appropriate-payment-approach/30838

NIHR guidance on payment to contributors: www.nihr.ac.uk/documents/payment-guidance-for-researchers-and-professionals/27392

NIHR INVOLVE resources including online evidence library: www.invo.org.uk/resource-centre/libraries

NIHR Research Design Service (RDS): www.nihr.ac.uk/explore-nihr/support/research-design-service.htm

NIHR Trial Steering Committee (TSC) guidance: www.nihr.ac.uk/documents/good-practice-guidelines-on-the-recruitment-and-involvement-of-public-members-on-trial-steering-committees-tscs-study-steering-committees-sscs/27-348

Peninsula Public Engagement Group (PenPEG) service user involvement group: https://arc-swp.nihr.ac.uk/patient-public-involvement-engagement/groups-we-work-with/penpeg/

PiiAF guidance: https://piiaf.org.uk/documents/piiaf-guidance-jan14.pdf

Reporting the Involvement of Patients and the Public (GRIPP): www.bmj.com/content/358/bmj.j3453

Reward and recognition for public contributors – a guide to the payment of fees and expenses: https://www.nihr.ac.uk/documents/reward-and-recognition-for-public-contributors-a-guide-to-the-payment-of-fees-and-expenses/12248

UK Standards pilot projects: https://sites.google.com/nihr.ac.uk/pi-standards/test-beds

UK Standards for public involvement: https://drive.google.com/file/d/1EZU3uWwdH36-B3idleKf0radZj5bBcOo/view

CHAPTER 6

Qualitative research

06

6.1 Introduction

6.1.1 What is qualitative research?

Qualitative research aims to provide an in-depth understanding of how people make sense of the world and experience events. It seeks to explain the 'how' and 'why' of behaviour and to gain insight into what it is like to be in someone else's shoes. It involves analysing non-numerical data (audio, video, photographs and text) and aims to study people in a natural setting.

6.1.2 Differences to quantitative research

Quantitative research sets out to test hypotheses based on previous evidence (known as a **deductive** process). It requires a large randomly selected sample to increase the generalisability of findings. This type of research produces numerical data which is analysed using statistical methods and follows a linear process, working through a pre-determined protocol to reduce bias.

Conversely, qualitative research does not test hypotheses but instead aims to generate hypotheses. This is known as an **inductive** process, whereby theory is created from data with no preconceived ideas. This means it falls under the realm of exploratory research as described in *Section 3.9.1*. It uses a much smaller sample size to provide rich data which is described in words and does not use statistics in data analysis. It is interpretative, meaning it seeks to explain the underlying reasons/motivations behind a phenomenon. Furthermore, qualitative research employs an **iterative** approach, which means that the methodology can be refined throughout the study based on what has been found so far. This can help generate more useful and high-quality data; for instance, if a researcher was conducting interviews and found that a particular question elicited a lot of interesting data, the methodology for future interviews may be adapted to focus more on this topic area.

This is summarised in *Table 6.1*.

Table 6.1: Summary of the differences between quantitative and qualitative research approaches

Quantitative research	Qualitative research
Numerical data	Non-numerical data
Tests hypotheses (deductive)	Generates hypothesis (inductive)
More generalisable	Not generalisable
Large sample size	Small sample size
Statistical analysis	Does not use statistics
Summarised in numbers	Summarised in words
Pre-determined protocol	Iterative
Descriptive ('what')	Interpretative ('why')

6.1.3 When might you use it?

Because qualitative analysis provides detailed data, it can retain complexities and uncover subtleties that are often missed by quantitative analysis. Qualitative studies are humanistic and aim for an empathetic interpretation. This means we can use them to provide insight into patients' perspectives.

You may want to employ a qualitative research method within a clinical research setting to investigate:

- motivations underlying health behaviour
- patients' experiences of interventions
- healthcare workers' perspectives on running of services
- patients' perceptions about healthcare access
- healthcare workers' perspectives on the implementation of new practices.

Whether a quantitative or qualitative approach is best depends on your research question. Examples of questions which may suit each approach are listed in *Table 6.2*.

Table 6.2: Examples of qualitative and quantitative research questions

Quantitative research	Qualitative research
When should rheumatoid arthritis patients be switched to a different biological therapy if they are not responding?	What are the experiences of rheumatoid arthritis patients accessing NHS care in London?
Which is the most effective treatment for the negative symptoms of schizophrenia?	Why do some people with schizophrenia not adhere to treatment?
What biomarkers predict treatment response to depression therapies?	How do patients with depression feel about biomarker testing?
What is the effect of pregabalin on visual analogue pain score?	What does a reduction in a score of 2 on visual analogue mean from a patient's perspective?

6.1.4 Philosophical positions

Philosophical positions provide principles of theoretical thinking which are used to make assumptions while conducting qualitative research, so it is important to understand these to be able to interpret findings in a meaningful way. **Ontology** is the study of reality, or what there is to know about. **Epistemology** is the study of knowledge, or how reality can be made known to us. Philosophical positions can help us to understand the differences between quantitative and qualitative research. Quantitative research takes a **positivist position** which states that there is a single objective reality which can be discovered through appropriate observational methods. Qualitative research tends to draw on a **constructivist position** which states that there are multiple realities which are created by each individual through interpreting the world around them. This is summarised in *Table 6.3*.

Table 6.3: Summary of philosophical positions

	Positivist position (quantitative)	Constructivist position (qualitative)
Ontology	There is one objective reality	Reality is socially constructed
		There are multiple realities/perspectives
Epistemology	Knowledge can be gained by what is directly observed by the senses	Knowledge can be gained by understanding the multiple views of people in a particular context
		The researcher's subjective influence on interpretation must be considered

6.1.5 Ethical considerations

If the nature of the study is a sensitive topic, psychological harm needs to be considered. During interviews on a sensitive topic participants may have to revisit painful memories which could cause emotional distress. In this case the researcher must ensure that they can refer participants to a counselling service.

Participants must be informed about the aim of the study, whether it will be recorded, and reminded that their participation is voluntary and that they do not have to answer questions that they don't feel comfortable with. The researcher must explain that their data will be kept confidential, and that their identity will be kept anonymous; for example, audio and video recordings will be deleted after transcription and all identifying characteristics are removed from the transcripts. The participant is then asked for verbal informed consent. This is covered in more detail in *Section 4.5.1*.

6.1.6 Disadvantages

The main drawbacks to qualitative research are that it is not generalisable to the population; however, this does not mean that the findings are not valuable. Qualitative research aims to understand personal experiences in a specific context, which cannot be captured through traditional quantitative measures.

Another disadvantage is that collecting and analysing qualitative data is very time-consuming. For instance, in-depth interviews may take over an hour to conduct and transcribing the audio recording can take over 5 hours per interview. Following this, data analysis can also be a lengthy process. Nevertheless, this is necessary to produce rich detailed data.

6.2   Sampling

As previously mentioned, qualitative research selects small samples via non-probability sampling (where the likelihood of being selected in the sample is unknown), thus the sample is not representative of the population. Despite this, much consideration goes into selecting participants so that they are rich with data and insights. For instance, participants may be sought who have personal experiences of a certain treatment regime, or a diverse sample may be chosen to gain a wide range of perspectives. Below are common sampling methods in qualitative research. You may recall convenience sampling mentioned in *Section 3.2.2*.

6.2.1 Types of sampling in qualitative research

Purposive sampling

This relies on the researcher's judgement on who should be included in the study to obtain a sample which they think will provide the most insights into their research question. For instance, in a study investigating the barriers to quitting smoking, researchers may decide to enrol people of a variety of ages, years smoking, and pharmacotherapies to get a diverse range of views on the topic. This is known as heterogeneous or maximum variation sampling.

Quota sampling

This is similar to purposive sampling but the desired characteristics of the sample are chosen beforehand and a target quota is given for each subgroup. For instance, researchers may decide they want five women, five men, three people aged under 30, three people aged over 60, etc.

Snowball sampling

This involves asking participants to recommend other people they know to be included in the study (who meet the inclusion criteria). This is not likely to be representative of a population; however, it can be useful when trying to reach hard-to-reach communities such as those who do not readily engage with research / healthcare services.

Convenience sampling

As discussed in *Section 3.2.2* this involves recruiting participants in a way that is convenient; for example, through networks within an organisation. It is an easy way to recruit a large number of participants but it may not provide a diverse set of viewpoints so it is most useful in initial exploratory research.

6.2.2 Data saturation

This is the point at which no new concepts emerge from your data. After this has been reached, recruitment can cease and your sample size is considered large enough.

6.3 Data collection methods

6.3.1 Documentary evidence

This uses data from a secondary resource such as data from medical records, support groups, social media and blog posts, newspaper articles, school reports and diaries. The advantage of this method is it does not require resources to collect data as it utilises data that is already available. This can be especially useful for historical research; for instance, how treatments for a disease have developed over time. The main disadvantages of this method are that we need to be wary about the credibility and authenticity of sources. It can be hard to determine whether this data is an accurate representation of the person's perspective and what the motives were for writing the source; for instance, a news article may be biased by external sponsorship.

6.3.2 Surveys

Qualitative surveys or questionnaires contain open-ended questions where respondents may be prompted to provide longer answers. These can yield more detailed information than multiple choice or rating scale style questions and can provide reasoning behind answers to other questions. The downside of surveys is that they are very structured and do not offer the researcher a chance to probe the respondent for more information; however, they are easily administered and recruited for, especially if they use an online platform. They can also serve as an ideal starting point to identify topics of interest to investigate further using other methods.

6.3.3 Interviews

These are one-on-one discussions between a researcher and a participant which generate detailed individual-level data through discussions on a particular topic (see *Figure 6.1* for additional information). During this process the researcher will ask questions to encourage the participant to share their perspective and experience. These can generate detailed data and a deep understanding of a topic, especially when not much is known about an area. They are also useful for studying sensitive topics which participants may not feel comfortable talking about in a group setting such as a focus group. Interviews can vary in length but tend to be around 20–60 minutes each.

Increasing depth

Structured	Pre-determined questions are administered verbally with little to no flexibility to deviate from these. This may be useful if questions need to be clarified or participants have literacy problems.
Semi-structured	These use a topic guide, which is a list of key questions and topics to be explored in the interview. However, the interviewee may diverge from this and ask follow-up questions in order to explore an area in greater detail. This format is most commonly used by healthcare researchers.
Unstructured	These have few to no pre-determined topics or questions to cover. The interviewer may ask an opening question to begin the interview and then decide to explore different areas based on the interviewees' answers. These are ideal when little is known about an area and considerable depth is desired.

Less time required

Figure 6.1. Summary of interview structures.

Topic guide

A **topic guide** is used for reference to guide the discussion and maintain consistency across interviews. It contains the key questions about the topic of interest. It is advisable to familiarise yourself with the guide so that you can focus solely on the interviewee. Although it contains important questions, it should not be seen as a formal script, and it should be structured in a way that naturally flows. It may be useful to pilot the topic guide with colleagues or an initial group of interviewees to see if it flows smoothly, if questions are easy to understand, and if it is able to yield detailed answers. The initial group of interviewees may also draw attention to new areas of importance which were not previously thought about by the research team, causing the topic guide to be refined.

Recording

It is advised to record interviews as this produces the most accurate data and is not biased by memory. Most commonly, this is then transcribed verbatim, i.e. word for word. **Field notes** should also be recorded which are reflections on the interview, the environment, the body language of the participant as well as anything that was said after the recording stopped.

Conducting the interview

A quiet and private location free from distractions should be chosen. The effect of the settings on the participant must also be considered; for instance, the choice of a clinical setting could create a perception of power imbalance due to the participant adopting the patient role.

Interview Timeline

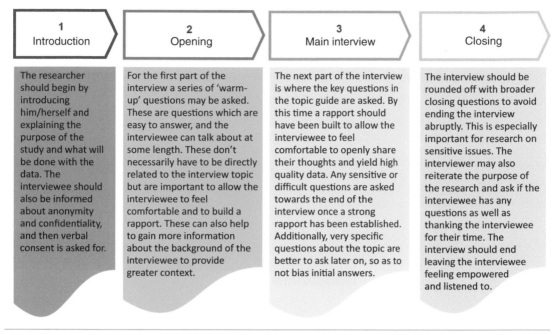

1 Introduction	2 Opening	3 Main interview	4 Closing
The researcher should begin by introducing him/herself and explaining the purpose of the study and what will be done with the data. The interviewee should also be informed about anonymity and confidentiality, and then verbal consent is asked for.	For the first part of the interview a series of 'warm-up' questions may be asked. These are questions which are easy to answer, and the interviewee can talk about at some length. These don't necessarily have to be directly related to the interview topic but are important to allow the interviewee to feel comfortable and to build a rapport. These can also help to gain more information about the background of the interviewee to provide greater context.	The next part of the interview is where the key questions in the topic guide are asked. By this time a rapport should have been built to allow the interviewee to feel comfortable to openly share their thoughts and yield high quality data. Any sensitive or difficult questions are asked towards the end of the interview once a strong rapport has been established. Additionally, very specific questions about the topic are better to ask later on, so as to not bias initial answers.	The interview should be rounded off with broader closing questions to avoid ending the interview abruptly. This is especially important for research on sensitive issues. The interviewer may also reiterate the purpose of the research and ask if the interviewee has any questions as well as thanking the interviewee for their time. The interview should end leaving the interviewee feeling empowered and listened to.

Figure 6.2. Diagram showing the timeline of an interview.

Perfecting interview technique is a skill which takes practice (see *Figure 6.2*). The aim is to encourage the interviewee to answer the questions as honestly and thoroughly as possible. Therefore, good social skills are necessary to build a rapport with the interviewee by being empathetic, open, engaged and non-judgemental. A good way to do this is by using active listening techniques such as paraphrasing what the interviewee said, nodding, and using exclamations like 'Mmm', 'Wow!', 'That must have been difficult' and 'That's interesting'.

The interviewer should probe the interviewee with follow-up questions like 'What do you mean when you say…?' throughout the interview to get further clarification on topics and control the interview direction; for example, to steer back to the research topic if the interviewee has gone off on a tangent. It is also important to get the correct balance between the amount of talking and listening as too little talking will lead to a passive interview which may not stay on topic, and too much will not allow the interviewee enough time to finish their answers and may leave them wondering if they are providing the right information. Finally, a good interviewer should be able to challenge the interviewee and ask for clarification if they are answering inconsistently.

How to ask good questions

Questions which can be answered with one word should be avoided and instead questions which can elicit a long response should be used. Questions should be kept simple, and jargon should be avoided.

What to avoid

Below are a series of question types that should be avoided.

Leading: I suppose you think it's difficult to make appointments at your GP surgery?	**Alternative:** How do you feel about making appointments at your GP surgery?
Too insensitive: I bet you were really upset when you found out?	**Alternative:** Can you describe the day you got your diagnosis; how did you feel when you first found out?
Too vague: What is it like having osteoarthritis?	**Alternative:** How does having osteoarthritis affect your daily activities?
Biased: Do you think the urgent need to reduce obesity is adequately reported in the media?	**Alternative:** What do you think about the media coverage on obesity?
Double negative: Do you think people should stop not seeking help for health problems?	**Alternative:** Do you think people should seek help for health problems?
Multiple-barrelled: How severe are your symptoms? Do you take any medications?	

WORKED EXAMPLE
GPs' perceptions of workload in England: a qualitative interview study

Croxson *et al.*, (2017) *Br J Gen Pract*, 67: e138, doi.org/10.3399/bjgp17X688849

Background

This study aimed to gain an understanding of UK NHS GPs' perceptions about workload.

Methods

Participants were recruited by advertisements sent via regional GP email lists and social media networks in June 2015. Responses were received from 171 GPs, and 34 were selected to participate in this study based on GP characteristics (sessions per week, years as a GP, additional roles, GP role) and practice characteristics (list size, geographical location, rurality, number of other staff) to obtain a maximum-variation sample. Semi-structured interviews were conducted between June and July 2015, either face-to-face or via telephone by an independent research team comprising clinical and non-clinical researchers. Interviews lasted between 30 and 70 minutes and participants provided oral or written consent. Interviews were audio recorded, transcribed verbatim, and anonymised.

Comments

- This is an example of purposive sampling. As all the GPs working in NHS England were eligible and advertisements were sent through region lists, the study team were able to gain a large sample from which to select a variety of GP characteristics, thereby capturing a wide range of perspectives. The downsides to the approach used are that the interviews were conducted during the summer months, and responses may have been different during winter months which are busier. Also, GPs who felt strongly about workload would be more likely to volunteer, possibly resulting in over-reporting of workload issues.

- As the interviews were conducted by a non-GP, participants may have felt able to speak openly about their feelings. Interviews are ideal for this study as it is investigating individual-level perspectives.

Topic guide

- Can you describe your workload? (volume, working hours, intensity)
- Can you describe a typical working day/week?
- How do you feel about your workload? (manageability, sustainability, job satisfaction)
- What contributes to your workload? (patient care, other activities)
- Do you think that your workload has changed over time? (when, why, how)
- What are your thoughts about the content of consultations? (complexity, duration, change over time, what makes consultations complex)
- How is workload distributed across your practice?
- What factors influence your workload?
- How do you cope with your workload?
- Do you/your practice have any strategies for dealing with the workload? (how effective do you think these strategies are?)
- Do you have any ideas for other strategies for dealing with the workload?
- Are you expecting workload to change in the future?
- Is there anything else about GP workload that you'd like to mention?

Comments

- The topic guide was produced by reviewing existing literature combined with discussions with GPs and the research team.
- An academic GP conducted pilot interviews and the topic guide was amended following these. The topic guide was amended further throughout the study. This is an example of the iterative nature of qualitative research.

Results

The findings of this study were consistent with surveys and quantitative assessments of consultation rates. Four major themes emerged to explain the increase in workload: increasing patient needs/expectations, the changing relationship between primary and secondary care, bureaucracy and resources, and the workload balance within practices.

Example of findings from one of the themes:

Patients' needs and expectations

Some GPs felt that there was diminishing self-management due to:

Less social support from the community

"I think we are the first port of call when somebody's relationship goes wrong or somebody loses their job, or whatever it is, and that takes time because often there isn't anything medically wrong with them … just people who've had something bad happen. There just isn't the social support in the community, and so we are the port of call for that, and that probably has had some increase."

As well as increasing access to health information online, along with public health media campaigns:

"The media campaigns, you know: 'Go and see your doctor if you've had a cough for 3 weeks', that kind of thing ... all of a sudden everybody with a cough for 3 weeks during 'flu season comes in. So yes, so health campaigns affect workload, local health scares."

Many participants attributed higher workload to being situated in more deprived areas where patients were less educated about health and requested more consultations for minor illnesses:

"Quite a large cohort of homeless people, street workers, and drug substance abuse that actually take a long time to obviously sort out and the constraints of the 10 minutes, it's pretty much impossible to sort of sort that out. Whereas my rural practice ... the patients around here are a lot more affluent and there's a lot of worried well, so a lot of consultations where perhaps not as much health care has happened that I'd expected to, and the sort of demands are sometimes unreasonable."

> **Comments**
> * These excerpts give a sense of the detailed data you can gain from interviews to obtain a more nuanced and in-depth understanding of how the multiple factors identified in quantitative studies may be contributing to increased workload. These findings are particularly useful for informing decisions on strategies addressing this.

6.3.4 Focus groups

These are discussions between the researcher and a small group of participants on a specific topic. Like interviews, they can gather data on participants' perspectives but are able to obtain a broad range of views in one go and understand how these topics may be discussed in a group. For instance, controversial issues may be uncovered, and debates may prompt participants to rationalise their comments, which can help us to understand the meaning behind different viewpoints.

Choosing the group

Group composition and its effect on the discussion must be carefully considered. Pre-existing groups may be chosen as they can be easier to recruit and participants may feel comfortable around each other, which facilitates open discussions. On the other hand, stranger groups may be chosen to gather different viewpoints from people with a variety of socio-demographic characteristics. Participants in stranger groups may also feel more comfortable due to greater anonymity, allowing them to freely express opinions which they would not share in a pre-existing group that shares a different viewpoint. A focus group which contains people with varying educational and economic statuses may create a sense of hierarchy, causing some participants to feel more reserved. Another possible group set-up is running different sessions with groups of people with similar characteristics, e.g. a female-only group. This may help participants feel more comfortable and allows for clustering of findings for different types of participants.

A group size of six to eight participants is recommended as this allows for a range of opinions but is small enough to give everyone a chance to speak; however, larger discussion groups are possible. It is better to recruit too many participants to allow for cancellations, but smaller groups are suitable when the participants are very knowledgeable about the subject.

Conducting the focus group

The **moderator** is responsible for guiding the discussion through a set of topics. They must be able to keep the discussion focused and on topic, but not join the discussion (as this introduces bias) and ensure that all participants are given an equal chance to speak, i.e. the discussion is not being dominated by one person. As with interviews, it is important to remain non-judgemental and have open and neutral body language (even if views are expressed which the moderator personally disagrees with).

The general conduct is similar to interviews, whereby the moderator will introduce themself and the research aims and gain verbal consent for participation and audio recordings. Again, they will begin by asking opening questions to build up a rapport, probe for additional information and ask the more sensitive questions towards the end. As with interviews, the setting should be carefully considered to ensure the participants are comfortable and that background noise will be kept to a minimum to ensure the recording can be heard clearly. There may also be a note-taker present who is responsible for writing filed notes and will serve as a backup if the recording fails.

Probing examples:

"Sameer has made an interesting comment, does anyone else have a similar/different opinion?"

"There are several different views being expressed, can anyone explain the reasoning behind their opinions?"

"I can see you are nodding Terry; do you agree with Sameer?"

"Daniella we also value your opinion, do you have anything to add?"

WORKED EXAMPLE
Barriers to uptake and adherence with malaria prophylaxis by the African community in London, England: focus group study

Morgan and Figueroa-Muñoz (2007) *Ethnicity & Health*, **10**: 355, doi.org/10.1080/13557850500242035

Background

This study aimed to investigate beliefs surrounding uptake of and adherence to malaria prophylaxis in individuals of African descent in inner London.

Methods

Focus groups were held in a community centre with 44 volunteers of African origin to explore views about malaria prophylaxis among the African community.

> **Comments**
> - As this is an exploratory study, focus groups are an ideal approach as they can uncover a wide variety of views and topics quickly which may be unknown to researchers. Conversations about non-adherence may be sustained better in a group setting compared to a one-to-one interview, and focus groups are ideal for studies on views held by ethnic minorities as they investigate group views. Additionally, this topic is not sensitive or embarrassing so is not inappropriate to discuss among a group.

Local church and community workers from the African community were encouraged to help with recruiting volunteers as they knew a wide range of people of West African origin. It was emphasised that the group should include people with a mix of socio-demographic characteristics. Motivations for attendance were also mixed: some volunteers saw the groups as a social event and others had a strong interest in malaria.

> **Comments**
> - This is an example of a snowball sample. This approach successfully recruited a diverse sample in terms of age, education and occupation to identify a range of beliefs.

Meetings began with a hot buffet of African foods where participants could meet informally.

> **Comments**
> - The setting was chosen to create an informal and welcoming atmosphere which helps build rapport between members of the group.

The sessions began with participants describing their experiences of having malaria. This stimulated discussion with members of the group comparing experiences and identified several issues that were not originally identified by the research agenda. These were then probed by the facilitator; for example, use and views of traditional medicine.

> **Comments**
> - This demonstrates the use of an 'ice-breaker' activity to begin the focus group and stimulate initial discussions in the group.

After five focus groups the main themes were recurring, so no more sessions were held.

> **Comments**
> - The researcher chose to hold several repeating focus groups until reaching data saturation, whereby holding more sessions is unlikely to add more material. This indicates that the data collection is adequate for examining this topic.

The participants were made aware of the fact that the main facilitator was a public health doctor from an ethnic minority background whose interest in malaria stemmed from their own experience of living in tropical countries. The correctness of viewpoints was not discussed.

Comments

- The facilitator was aware of the possible influence of how they were perceived by the group on the data generated, and made an effort to establish commonality and a non-judgemental environment to encourage open discussions.
- Focus groups also provide a supportive environment due to being surrounded by other members of the community; this can address issues of perceived power which may occur in interview situations.

Results

There was substantial variability in the viewpoints held by different members of the group. People who held professional occupations had greater knowledge of the different types of drugs and issues such as waning immunity, through accessing information online. On the other hand, participants with occupations that suggested a lower education level had beliefs that they were not at risk or were already vaccinated (at a time when no vaccine existed). This group also tended to return to visit family members living in poorer rural communities in Africa where prevalence rates are higher.

Comments

- Focus groups with diverse samples can allow us to interpret how socioeconomic characteristics may feed into different beliefs, which could form the basis of more research examining this more rigorously.

Respondents generally agreed that household leaflets were not likely to be read and that health promotion messages regarding prophylaxis would have more engagement through using local radio stations, churches and community venues involving community leaders.

Comments

- This is useful information for implementation of public health campaigns to increase prophylaxis adherence.

6.3.5 Observational studies

This is a method whereby the researcher systematically observes and records people's behaviour in their natural settings. Qualitative observational studies differ from observational epistemology studies mentioned in *Section 2.6* and clinical observations of a patient. The main advantage of observation is that it can identify the discrepancies between what people say and their actions. These can occur due to difficulties recalling memories, fear of judgement or people simply not being aware of their behaviours. It can also be used in conjunction with other types of qualitative methods, such as interviews, to provide a more complete picture.

The main types of observation are outlined below:

Participant observation – the researcher takes part in the activities that they are observing and must develop a rapport with the group being observed. The degree of participation will vary depending on the research area; however, the presence of the researcher may change how the people being observed act.

Non-participant observation – the researcher observes people or activities from a distance without being involved. This also includes covert observation, which is less common as it poses ethical considerations but may be appropriate in some settings.

Visual aided observation – this is observation with the use of video equipment. This is commonly used when the presence of the researcher would heavily impact the interactions or be very intrusive, such as observing a counselling session. The researcher must gain informed consent beforehand.

Recording

The field notes gathered during observations become the data for analysis, so these must be clear and detailed. These may include descriptions of the setting, smells and sounds of a place, and the interactions between people, including body language, expressions and conversations. A researcher may also keep a field diary which can contain how the researcher felt and reacted to a situation and their interpretations of what they observed.

WORKED EXAMPLE
Room design – a phenomenological-hermeneutical study

Sundberg *et al.* (2019), *Crit Care Nurs Q*, **42**: 265, doi.org/10.1097/CNQ.0000000000000267

Background

This study investigated the effects of evidence-based redesign of the ICU room environment on caring attitudes of nursing staff in a Swedish hospital.

Methods

This involved ten non-participant observations of two different room designs and was followed by interviews with the nurses. These observations were carried out by one researcher who was an experienced ICU nurse but who had not worked in the research setting.

> Comments
> * The observer in this study was an 'insider', meaning she had shared experiences and characteristics with those being observed. This was an advantage as she possessed the theoretical sensitivity needed for detailed data collection and critical analysis. This meant she could also change from a non-participant observer to a participant observer if an incident required her to act. However, as the staff were aware of the researcher's professional identity this could have affected how they acted.

- Relationships between staff and researchers were established prior to the study through previous research studies as well as seminars given by the research team to the ICU nurses. This ensured the nurses fully understood the purpose of the study and enabled access to the ICU to be established by the researcher.

The researcher sat quietly in the corner of the room and wore the same scrubs as the nurses. Each observation was centred around a critical care nurse and assistant nurse. Fifteen staff were observed in total with a range of ages (22–55) and work experience (between 3 weeks and 12 years). The older room design was observed to begin with, to act as a control for baseline observations. A total of 47.5 hours of observations were made across both daytime and evening shifts, which were documented in hand-written descriptive and reflective field notes.

Comments

- The researcher wore the same scrubs as staff to comply with hygiene standards and to blend into the environment. The researcher chose to write hand-written field notes to reduce intrusion.

Ethics

Research ethics committee approval was gained, and written and oral information was provided to the staff about the study at its onset and during staff meetings. However, the specific focus of the observations was not disclosed, in order not to bias the staff's actions. The voluntary nature of participation, confidentiality and right to decline were emphasised so that staff who did not wish to participate could choose to work in rooms which were not being observed. Critically ill patients are considered vulnerable research participants who require thorough ethical consideration. Due to their background, the researchers were conscious of the vulnerabilities of ICU patients and family distress so could withdraw observation when appropriate. The next of kin were not required to give informed consent on behalf of the patients in this study, as this is not required under the Swedish research ethics regulations. If observations were carried out when patients were awake the researcher would explain the reason for her presence and obtain informed consent. It was emphasised that the observation was focused on nursing activities and would not affect patient care. The researcher did not attend handover reports where personal information was shared.

Comments

- In the UK informed consent from next of kin would be required for this study, so it is important to adhere to ethical guidelines in the country where the study is taking place. This highlights the ethical considerations when carrying out an observation in an environment with vulnerable patients, and the way in which this can be carried out appropriately and sensitively with minimal intrusion.

Link to additional analysis of this study

Qualitative observational research in the intensive care setting: a personal reflection on navigating ethical and methodological issues

Sundberg *et al.* (2021), *INQUIRY: J Health Care Org, Prov and Finance*, **58**: doi.org/10.1177/00469580211060299

6.3.6 **Mixed methods**

This involves combining qualitative and quantitative methods to investigate a research question. This could be useful to explore the reasoning behind responses and create a more nuanced picture of data from quantitative measures. On the other hand, quantitative studies may increase generalisability of findings from qualitative findings. The downsides of this approach are that it is the most labour-intensive, and it can be challenging to interpret conflicting results.

Examples:

- How do clinic waiting times (quantitative) affect reports of patient satisfaction (qualitative)?
- How do patient beliefs (qualitative) help to explain adherence to drug therapy (quantitative)?
- How do anxiety and depression scores (quantitative) compare with patients' experiences of pain (qualitative)?

Table 6.4 summarises the qualitative approaches we have discussed in this section.

Table 6.4: Summary of key methods in qualitative research

Approach	Advantages	Disadvantages
Qualitative interview	Useful for discussing sensitive or embarrassing topics Useful to gain rich data where considerable depth is required	Can be very time-intensive Power imbalance may be perceived by the interviewee
Focus groups	Useful for investigating views held by a community The group dynamic can encourage more discussion and rationalisation of viewpoints Wide range of views obtained in one go	Group dynamics can prevent some participants from sharing their views freely Not useful for investigating individual-level perspectives Not suitable for discussing sensitive issues
Observation	Can highlight inconsistencies between what people say and what they do Can be used in combination with other methods to gain a more holistic picture	The observer is making interpretations about what they are viewing Participants may act differently if they know they are being observed, and non-participant observation may pose ethical concerns

6.4   Analysis

Before beginning your qualitative research study, you will decide on the type of analysis method you wish to use. Which approach is most appropriate will depend on your research question and epistemological perspective, since each approach provides a different way of thinking about the data based on assumptions and theoretical frameworks. Qualitative analysis occurs during data collection, as opposed to after with quantitative analysis. This is known as an iterative or cyclical process because findings from initial analysis will shape how the data is collected.

Table 6.5 summarises key qualitative data analysis methods and approaches.

Table 6.5: Summary of common qualitative data analysis approaches

Analysis method/ approach	Description	Applications
Content analysis	Strategies which use a systematic coding and categorising approach to find themes within a dataset	Quantify codes and describe the presence of patterns, meanings, and relationships or themes in a dataset
Thematic analysis	Identifies, analyses and interprets patterns or themes within a dataset	Finds patterns of meaning in a dataset in relation to a research topic and can be applied across a range of theoretical and epistemological positions
Grounded theory	Develops theories based on the iterative collection of data	Develop theories which are tightly linked with real-world data when there are no existing theories to explain the phenomena
Discourse analysis	Linguistic analysis of the flow of communication within its social, cultural or political context	Gain insights into how language is used and how meaning is constructed in different contexts, e.g. doctor–patient communications or health promotion messages
Narrative analysis	Aims to understand how people construct stories and narratives from personal experiences	Understanding how someone's chain of experiences have led them to their current state and how people make sense of their life by encoding it into a narrative
Interpretative phenomenological analysis (IPA)	Aims to understand how subjects experience the world within a particular context (phenomenon)	Understanding personal perceptions of a life event such as clinical diagnosis through a subject-centred perspective

Common techniques in data analysis

Most qualitative analysis approaches involve firstly organising data by transcribing interviews or focus group recordings or typing up field notes, followed by coding. **Coding** is a way of breaking down the data into categories and then assigning labels to these. This is a way to organise the data in a structured manner to identify themes and find relationships between them. Coding approaches may be deductive (top-down), meaning the researcher begins with a set of predetermined codes and then finds excerpts that fit those codes, or inductive (bottom-up), meaning the researcher derives codes from the data.

Computer-assisted qualitative data analysis software (CAQDAS)

Software is available to speed up processes such as transcription of interviews and can help with storing and organising codes. For virtual interviews, Microsoft Teams and

Zoom have built-in transcription services during recording. For other recordings, there are online services such as OTranscribe and Otter. After using one of these tools the researcher will still need to listen to the recording to check that the transcription has been accurate. One of the most popular CAQDAS is NVivo which helps organise codes, make analysis notes, quantify frequencies of codes, and identify relationships within the data.

In the next section we will discuss two of the most common forms of qualitative analysis for healthcare research in more detail: thematic analysis and grounded theory.

6.4.1 Thematic analysis

This is a good first qualitative analysis method to learn, as it provides useful skills for conducting other forms of analysis. It is similar to content analysis but instead of describing and quantifying codes it aims to be more interpretative. Braun and Clarke laid out a framework for using this method in 2006.

Themes

A **theme** captures something important about how the data relates to the research question. It must represent a repeated pattern of some level or a meaning. The researcher's judgement is necessary to assess this as there are no set rules about what constitutes a theme, and the prevalence of the theme doesn't necessarily dictate its importance. There are two types of themes: semantic and latent. Semantic themes are surface-level meanings of the data, i.e. describing what the participant has said, and latent themes read between the lines and look for underlying ideas and assumptions which shape the data.

Thematic analysis can use a top-down deductive approach where themes are guided by the researcher's focus, or a bottom-up inductive approach that is guided by the data.

Steps

1. **Become familiar with the data** – re-read transcripts several times and make notes on initial impressions.

2. **Generate initial codes** – organise data in a systematic way. This could either involve line-by-line coding using an inductive approach or coding any text that captures something relevant to the research question.

3. **Search for themes** – group together codes into themes.

4. **Refine themes** – modify and develop the themes identified; this can involve assessing whether the data supports the themes, combining overlapping themes, organising theme hierarchy and eliminating themes.

5. **Define themes** – identify the essence of each theme and identify how they relate to each other; refine the overall story the analysis tells.

6. **Write up** – select vivid extract examples, relate the analysis to the research question and literature.

The benefits of thematic analysis are that it is a relatively straightforward form of analysis that is easy to apply. Additionally, it is flexible as it can be applied across a range of theoretical and epistemological positions as it is not tied to any theoretical framework (unlike other methods like narrative analysis, discourse analysis and grounded theory). However, some difficulty may arise when deciding where the themes start and end – analysis with lots of overlapping themes or themes that are too large constitutes poor analysis. In some cases of bad thematic analysis, the researcher may not go beyond paraphrasing what the participants have said or make interpretations which do not reflect the underlying data. Furthermore, since coding breaks up the accounts into small chunks, any narrative or context to the account may be lost with this method.

WORKED EXAMPLE
A qualitative exploration of post-primary educators' attitudes regarding the promotion of student wellbeing

Byrne and Carthy (2021), *Int J Qual Studies Health Well-being*, **16**: 1, doi.org/10.1080/17482631.2021.1946928

Background

This study aimed to examine post-primary school educators' attitudes with regard to promotion of student wellbeing.

Methods

Eleven semi-structured interviews were conducted with post-primary educators in Ireland. Data was analysed through an inductive reflexive thematic analysis approach.

> #### Comments
> - This is one of the many forms of thematic analysis. It's flexible as the researcher can change and remove codes as they work through the data and it emphasises the researcher's subjective experience in the interpretation of data.

Analysis – coding

An example of preliminary coding is shown in *Figure 6.3*:

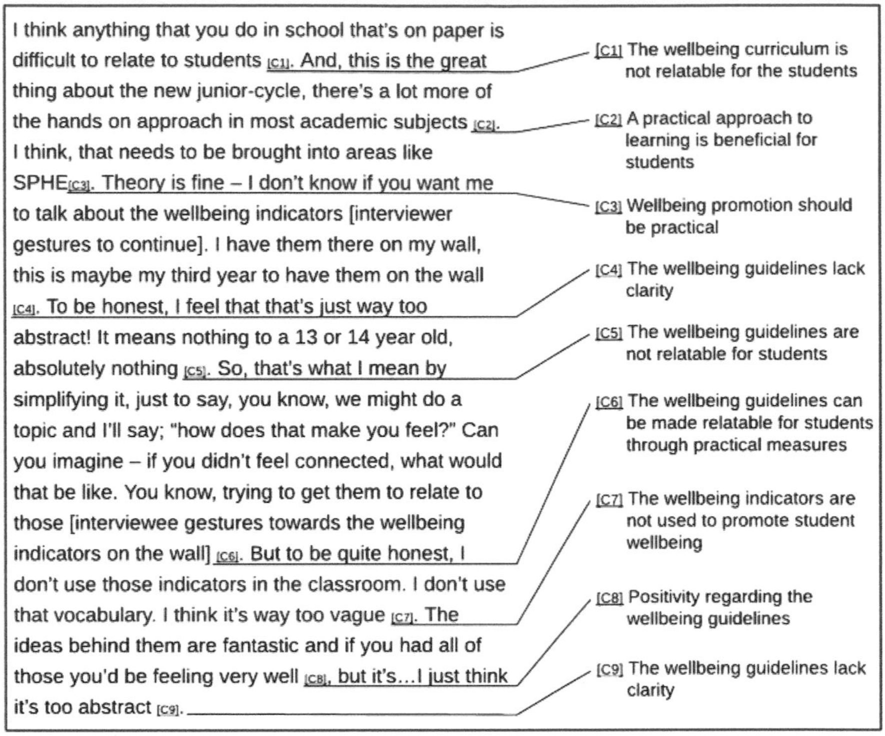

I think anything that you do in school that's on paper is difficult to relate to students [C1]. And, this is the great thing about the new junior-cycle, there's a lot more of the hands on approach in most academic subjects [C2]. I think, that needs to be brought into areas like SPHE[C3]. Theory is fine – I don't know if you want me to talk about the wellbeing indicators [interviewer gestures to continue]. I have them there on my wall, this is maybe my third year to have them on the wall [C4]. To be honest, I feel that that's just way too abstract! It means nothing to a 13 or 14 year old, absolutely nothing [C5]. So, that's what I mean by simplifying it, just to say, you know, we might do a topic and I'll say; "how does that make you feel?" Can you imagine – if you didn't feel connected, what would that be like. You know, trying to get them to relate to those [interviewee gestures towards the wellbeing indicators on the wall] [C6]. But to be quite honest, I don't use those indicators in the classroom. I don't use that vocabulary. I think it's way too vague [C7]. The ideas behind them are fantastic and if you had all of those you'd be feeling very well [C8], but it's…I just think it's too abstract [C9].

[C1] The wellbeing curriculum is not relatable for the students

[C2] A practical approach to learning is beneficial for students

[C3] Wellbeing promotion should be practical

[C4] The wellbeing guidelines lack clarity

[C5] The wellbeing guidelines are not relatable for students

[C6] The wellbeing guidelines can be made relatable for students through practical measures

[C7] The wellbeing indicators are not used to promote student wellbeing

[C8] Positivity regarding the wellbeing guidelines

[C9] The wellbeing guidelines lack clarity

Figure 6.3. Example of generating initial codes from an interview transcript. Reproduced from: 'A worked example of Braun and Clarke's approach to reflexive thematic analysis'. *Quality & Quantity*, 2021; **56**, 1391, under a CC BY 4.0 licence.

Comments
- Codes are brief but offer enough context to be viewed later as stand-alone descriptions of the underlying data.
- Code prevalence can be identified by looking at the number of occurrences throughout the entire dataset. This may indicate a pattern which could identify a theme; for example, C4/C9 appears twice already in this short extract and this code was informative in the development of a theme.

Iterations of coding were documented in a spreadsheet as data was revised and codes were refined.

Comments
- This helps to track the evolution of codes and themes to aid transparency.

Generating themes

The coded data was reviewed to determine how codes may be combined due to shared meanings. If a code appeared to be an over-arching narrative in the data, it was identified as a theme. The theme 'best practice in wellbeing promotion' was identified and broken down into two sub-themes which emphasised the involvement of the entire school staff and the pursuit of practical measures to promote student wellbeing. The theme 'recognising student wellbeing' was recognised and contained two sub-themes: 'inhibiting student wellbeing' and 'improving student wellbeing'. This grouping of factors improving and inhibiting wellbeing was also used for 'recognising educator wellbeing'. The theme 'factors influencing wellbeing promotion' contained four separate sub-themes: 'lack of training', 'lack of time', 'lack of appropriate value for wellbeing promotion' and 'lack of knowledge of supporting wellbeing-related documents'.

> Comments
> - Bringing all the information together was useful at an early stage; however, the 'factors influencing wellbeing promotion' theme was considered too dense and incoherent so required further revision.

Refining themes

Relationships between the data items and codes that inform the themes were assessed to see if they were appropriate to inform the theme (level 1 review), and then the themes were reviewed to see if they inform the interpretation of the dataset and related to the research question (level 2 review).

During level 1 review revisiting the data resulted in the 'sources of negative affect' sub-theme being split into two new sub-themes: 'work-related negative affect' and 'the influence of wellbeing promotion'.

> Comments
> - After review it was found that the data did not reflect just one theme.

During level 2 review it was decided that 'factors inhibiting wellbeing promotion' should be changed to 'the influence of time'.

> Comments
> - The initial theme did not accurately represent the data. The new theme recognised that previously existing time constraints affected wellbeing promotion.

Sub-themes 'lack of training' and 'knowledge of necessary documents' were collapsed into 'incompletely theorised agreements'.

> Comments
> - Coded items were found to create one narrative of educators not engaging with guidelines for wellbeing.

Level 2 review led to 'lack of value of wellbeing promotion' being changed to 'the value of wellbeing'.

> Comments
> - The initial theme was too simplistic, and it was realised that educators' perceptions of wellbeing promotion were not necessarily negative.

The final thematic map is shown in *Figure 6.4.*

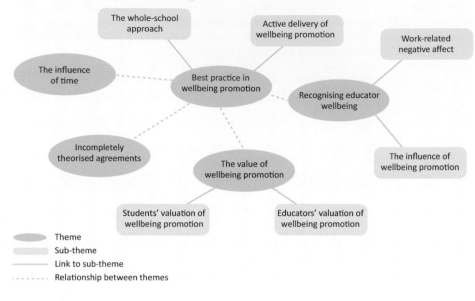

Figure 6.4. Final thematic map showing how themes and sub-themes interlink.

6.4.2 **Grounded theory**

Grounded theory (see *Figure 6.5*) was developed by Glaser and Strauss in 1967 to develop new theories based on the iterative collection of data. Therefore, the theory is 'grounded in data'. This is ideal when there is no existing theory for a phenomenon, or the existing theory has not been applied to a certain situation or population (as theoretical preconceptions should not be used). Firstly, data is collected from an initial group and analysed, then additional groups are examined to build upon the theory in order to endorse or refute data that has been previously identified; this is called theoretical sampling.

Memos are also recorded which explain thought patterns throughout data analysis and these are incorporated into the theory. Theoretical sampling ends when saturation has been reached.

The advantages of grounded theory are that findings are tightly linked with data, and as it does not use any preconceived hypotheses, it avoids confirmational bias. The downsides are that theoretical sampling is very labour-intensive, with the added difficulty of the inclusion criteria changing with each round of sampling. Additionally, constant comparisons may be hard with large amounts of data.

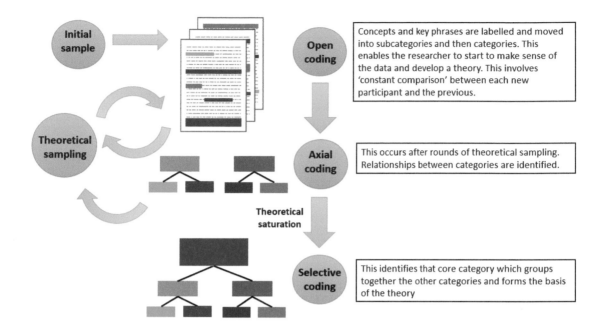

Figure 6.5. Stages of grounded theory.

WORKED EXAMPLE
Needing permission: the experience of self-care and self-compassion in nursing: a constructivist grounded theory study

Andrews *et al.* (2020), *Int J Nurs Stud*, **101**:103436, doi.org/10.1016/j.ijnurstu.2019.103436

Background

This study aimed to explore nurses' experience of self-care and self-compassion and investigate how this may relate to caregiving towards patients, using a grounded theory approach.

Methods

Semi-structured interviews lasting approximately 1 hour were conducted with nurses from two different NHS Trusts. Purposeful sampling was used to recruit general, mental health and learning disability nurses, at different levels of seniority. Theoretical sampling was used based on emerging data; for example, nurse leaders and newly qualified nurses were sought to expand on emerging categories. Data collection stopped after 30 nurses as saturation was reached. Interviews were recorded and transcribed verbatim, and initial line-by-line coding, axial coding and selective coding was performed, along with memo writing.

Example memo – 'Halcyon days of nursing'

"Halcyon days of nursing" – 22.03.16

Participant DQ2 spoke about the "halcyon days of nursing", during the 1980s, 1990s and early 2000s. On further discussion the changing NHS and culture was blamed on the move to a more business-like model.

Many of the participants reflected on the changing face of the NHS and nursing in general with many reasons for the changes being cited, including the above. Other changes featured the change in nurse training, negative healthcare enquiries with lessons learnt, changing management structures, more experienced staff leaving ward-based environments, a more threat-focused environment and the constant restructuring.

This will require further exploration as to whether there is any research looking at the changes in nursing or whether it is a more narrative experience at present. It seems to be a recurring theme throughout the data.

A link has also been made around not being able to have fun at work any more (participant RGN12). Why did this change? Have rules and guidance changed so much that staff feel unable to experience or have fun any more? Is this reality or perception?

"We gave ourselves permission to have fun and we don't do that anymore (no) and I don't think we're good at doing that with our teams as well" (RGN12)

Comments

- Here we can see the researchers using memos to start thinking about explanations for the data and record ideas about what needs to be explored further in the literature and in more subsequent rounds of theoretical sampling.

Results

Three concepts were derived from the data: 1) "hardwired to be caregivers", 2) needing a stable base, 3) managing the emotions of caring. These all linked to a core process: needing permission to self-care and be self-compassionate.

Comments

- *Figure 6.6* shows how analysis moved from surface-level description and summarising to interpretation to produce the three concepts that feed into the core concept.

Initial codes were developed to help give a sense of the data

Focused Codes	Categories	Core categories & Description	Concepts
		⇨ Theoretical Coding	
-Having no understanding of the key concepts -Role modelling as a precursor -Being unable to engage (Recognition not leading to action) -Being blocked -Needing to recognise and engage with the self -Learning process	-Training and experience -Background and early experience -Needing role models	<u>Motivating Factors</u> -The nursing story and background appears important – what motivated them to nurse and how does this relate to the nursing identity. -A focus on background, early experience and early role models appears key.	'Hardwired to be caregivers' Becoming and being a nurse (Are nurses hardwired to be caregivers? What is it about their story / journey that makes this so? Nurse as self versus nurse as professional role. These can be separate or more blurred depending on numerous internal and external factors. This appears related to the ability to give or receive permission in order to care for the self).
-Nursing character -Nursing Identity -Hardwired to be caregivers -Professional role / identity -Changing roles -Possessing and presenting certain characteristics -Fear of change -Feeling punished -Needing a sense of self	-Nurse as self -Nurse as a role -Nursing Character -Possessing compassion	<u>Nursing Identity</u> -Self-identity, and the factors involved in this awareness. -Possessing a particular nursing character with core values. -Is compassion innate or can it be learnt and nurtured as part of the nursing identity? -Identity as a fluid process. Nurse as self and nurse as role, with these appearing blurred at times and may change related to commitment to the organisation, how the nurse has been treated and whether they feel valued.	Giving self-permission (The ability to do this appears directly related to the factors involved with nursing identity and the motivations to nurse, including early messages, leading to accessibility and acceptability).

Figure 6.6. Example data showing the process of grounded theory. Reproduced with permission from Elsevier.

6.5   Conducting rigorous research

This section gives a brief overview of standards of rigour in qualitative research and suggested best practices throughout the design, data collection and analysis process to produce high-quality qualitative research.

6.5.1 Reflexivity

As the researcher is the primary instrument for data collection in qualitative research, they must be aware of how their social background, beliefs and assumptions can influence the data collected. **Reflexivity**, the process in which the researcher acknowledges their subjective influences on the research process, is therefore vital for rigorous research. This requires a great deal of self-awareness and reflection on the rationale behind decisions being made throughout the study. The reflective process must occur throughout every stage of the research process as the researcher's bias can affect all aspects of this, even during the inception of the research question. This concept can be exemplified by imagining a researcher who has lost a relative to lung cancer conducting a study on smoking habits; this personal experience could interfere with data collection or cause them to project their own views on analysis.

Qualitative research acknowledges that the researcher and the participant will contribute to the co-constructing data, therefore the researcher must acknowledge how their interpersonal dynamic can affect the data generated. This is known as interpersonal reflexivity. How the researcher is perceived by the interviewee may influence their answers; for instance, if a study was investigating anti-vaxxer beliefs and was conducted by a researcher dressed in scrubs, the interviewee may feel less able to be open about their beliefs.

6.5.2 Rigour throughout a study

Designing a study

As is true for embarking on any research endeavour, thorough review of the literature is required beforehand; this allows you to assess if your study is novel and advancing knowledge. The FINER approach is recommended to assess if the question is: **f**easible, **i**nteresting, **n**ovel, **e**thical and **r**elevant. In order to make the study feasible, the question should be specific, so the exact population and context should be defined. A strong conceptual framework must be constructed to justify the research question. However, since qualitative research uses an inductive approach, this framework should guide the questions and not dictate a hypothesis to be tested. When describing the chosen methods, the rationale behind the decision must be described.

Data collection

Data saturation is an important aspect of rigour to determine if sufficient data has been collected. Researchers should not only consider the number of participants but also the richness of data and quality of interviews to determine whether data with sufficient quality has been collected. For some studies with a narrower aim, interview quality may be more important to consider than quantity.

Prolonged engagement involves the researcher spending time to understand the context and culture of the person and situation being investigated, and is necessary to produce rich detailed data. Demonstrating an understanding of culture norms of the group being studied may also help to build a rapport between the participants and researcher.

Respondent validation or member checking is another standard of rigour which involves asking the participant to verify that the interview transcript is accurate and that the interpretation resonates with their experience.

Detailed records of raw data, field notes, transcripts and reflective journals can help with cross-referencing of data. **Audit trails** record the data collection process and rationale behind the decisions made throughout the study.

Use of purposeful or quota sampling is recommended where possible.

Triangulation is identifying convergences of data obtained using multiple methods or datasets to address a research question, and increases validity and rigour.

Other factors which may bias the study must be considered, e.g. method of recruitment, timing of the interview in relation to the experience being studied, the setting for an interview or focus group.

Data analysis

Stepwise replication should be carried out, which involves two researcher teams analysing data separately and then comparing and contrasting results.

Peer review involves inviting independent researchers to analyse the audit trails and critique the study methods and interpretations made by the researchers.

Negative case analysis is also important for maintaining rigour. This means actively finding and scrutinising data that contradicts the overall interpretation of the study, and using this to revise theoretical generalisations.

Using CAQDAS can increase rigour by helping to organise and manage large datasets and helping to calculate semi-quantitative descriptive statistics, identify negative cases and estimate intercoder reliability.

Publication

Sufficient data should be presented, e.g. quotes to allow the reader to see the relationship between the data and the interpretation. The participants' contributions can be semi-quantified, e.g. 'most of the participants said…'. There should be transparent reporting of possible biases and confounders.

Standards for Reporting Qualitative Research (SRQR) is a framework which consists of 21 items describing what should be reported in a qualitative research publication.

6.5.3 Lincoln and Guba's criteria

Lincoln and Guba (1986) created four criteria for assessing the trustworthiness of qualitative research. These are described in *Table 6.6* and make use of the strategies highlighted in bold above.

Table 6.6: Summary of Lincoln and Guba's criteria for assessing the trustworthiness of qualitative research

Rigour criteria	Definition	Implementation strategies
Credibility *Internal validity*	Confidence in the 'truth' of the results	Prolonged engagement Peer review Respondent validation Negative case analysis
Transferability *External validity*	Contextual information is provided so that the extent to which the results can apply to other contexts can be determined	Data saturation Purposeful sampling
Dependability *Reliability*	The reproducibility of the findings	Research process is clearly documented Stepwise replication Audit trails
Confirmability *Objectivity*	The results are based on information gathered from the participants and not researcher bias; this is established when credibility, transferability and dependability have been reached	Reflexivity Triangulation

6.6 Chapter summary

This chapter has introduced methodology in qualitative research and the way in which it differs from quantitative research (which you may be more familiar with). We have outlined the main data collection methods and analysis approaches, as well as standards of rigour to think about when conducting qualitative research. After reading this chapter you should have a greater understanding of how using a qualitative approach can be valuable in clinical research.

6.7 References and useful resources

Braun, V. and Clarke, V. (2006) Using thematic analysis in psychology. *Qualitative Research in Psychology*, 3: 77–101.

Glaser, B. and Strauss, A. (1967) *The Discovery of Grounded Theory: strategies for qualitative research*. Sociology Press.

Lincoln, Y.S. and Guba, E.G. (1986) But is it rigorous? Trustworthiness and authenticity in naturalistic evaluation. *N Dir Eval*, (30): 73–84.

O'Brien, B.C. *et al.* (2014) Standards for Reporting Qualitative Research: a synthesis of recommendations. *Acad Med*, 89(9): 1245–51.

CHAPTER 7

Disseminating your research findings

7.1 Introduction

Reporting and presenting findings from a research study is an important aspect of communication in research. It is important to report the findings of any research study in a timely and accurate manner. There are several considerations which need to be made, including adherence to guidelines for presenting data, e.g. from clinical trials, according to a CONSORT statement. Other studies such as genetic profiling analysis are also expected to be entered on databases where published data can then be accessed by readers, thereby adding to the body of literature that is available in a particular field.

7.1.1 Guidelines for presenting data based on study protocols

When reporting on data, it is important to adhere to the format and endpoints that were discussed in the original study protocol. Many clinical trials would be expected to be registered on databases, so that it is transparent from the time that the study is set up what the predetermined endpoints are for a particular study and what data is expected to be reported at the end of the study.

Many researchers will use international websites to enter information about their studies. For example, there are websites from the NHS providing information on clinical trials (www.nhs.uk/conditions/clinical-trials) and NIHR (National Institute for Health and Care Research) for UK-based studies (www.nihr.ac.uk). For specific conditions, e.g. cancer, there are websites that list current ongoing trials: www.cancerresearchuk.org/about-cancer/find-a-clinical-trial. Some countries have a legal requirement for researchers to register their trials and submit summary results (clinicaltrials.gov is the most commonly used example), which includes useful information including the published study protocol, the recruitment status of the study and eligibility criteria. There is also information provided such as study locations and staff contact information. At the end of the study, it is expected that a summary of the study is provided, including the baseline characteristics, outcome measures and adverse events.

7.1.2 **Guidelines for reporting different types of data**

There are a range of guidelines which need to be adhered to when reporting clinical studies and trials. The most widely used of these is the CONSORT guideline (www.consort-statement.org). Other guidelines that are commonly used include Cochrane recommendations for systematic reviews (https://training.cochrane.org/handbook) and PRISMA guidelines for systematic reviews and meta-analyses (www.prisma-statement.org). For further information see *Section 7.3.*

The reporting guidelines for CONSORT are summarised in *Table 7.1.*

Table 7.1: Summary of CONSORT reporting guidelines

CONSORT reporting guidelines	Information provided
Title	Informative title describing the study
Abstract	Summarise background, methods, results and discussion
Introduction	Explanation of the background, objectives and rationale for the study
Methods	Provide information on trial design, participants, eligibility criteria, settings, location of the study, interventions used in study, outcomes based on pre-specified primary and secondary outcome measures
	Include how and when participants were assessed, randomisation (with the methods used for this process), information about blinding for the study (e.g. single or double blind), participants, care providers, those assessing outcomes
	Statistics: describe groups compared, explain primary and secondary outcome measures
Results	Describe recruitment, baseline data, numbers analysed, outcomes and adverse effects
	A participant flow diagram is strongly recommended (see example in *Figure 7.1*)
Discussion	Describe study limitations, generalisability and interpretation

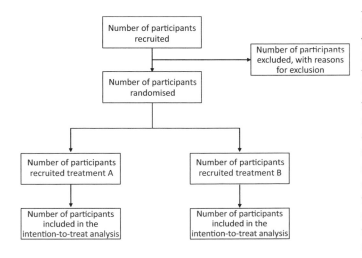

Figure 7.1. Sample study flow diagram. This example is for a clinical trial comparing two drugs: treatment A and B. It is best practice to report the number of participants recruited, the number excluded and reasons given (e.g. not suitable to take study drug), the number of subjects receiving each treatment, and the number of participants included in the intention-to-treat analysis (as shown in *Table 7.1*).

Databases for specific types of data

Many funders and publishers now expect authors to deposit data in recognised databases once it is completed so that the data is openly accessible to the research community, the funders and the public. If you are conducting laboratory-based studies, e.g. genome-wide association studies, with large datasets such as UK Biobank, it is useful for your data to be stored so as to be available for use in addressing future research questions and studies. Gene sequencing data can also be deposited in databases such as NCBI (National Centre for Biotechnology Information) and ArrayExpress. Other databases may be more disease-specific, e.g. the Cancer Genome Atlas. By depositing data, it can then be accessed by researchers in the field who may wish to ask research questions related to the initial findings or develop new projects, thereby adding to the body of scientific literature.

7.1.3 Funders

It is important to check the publishing policy with the funders of the project. For many funders, the preferred option is to publish in open access journals, which allows research to be accessible to other researchers, educators, members of the public and policy makers without added subscription charges or restrictions. Some funders will ask to share study data with them before publication. Certain funders will also contribute financially to open access charges, which can range from £500 to several thousand pounds, depending on the journal, and if colour illustrations are being used there may be an extra charge that journals stipulate. It is useful to clarify and request open access charges in grant applications with funders, if it is part of their policy, to assist in publication of research findings and ensure wide dissemination.

7.2 Poster presentations

When you have completed the main part of your data analysis, you may wish to present your data at a research conference in the field.

7.2.1 Where to start

When choosing an appropriate conference to present your work, it is important to establish the optimal audience for your research. This may be a society to which you belong, which may have a journal associated with it. The aim of presenting work at a conference, either as an oral presentation or a poster, is to outline, explain and discuss your research findings with a knowledgeable audience who have not seen your data before. If it is a completely novel piece of research, e.g. a clinical trial of a new drug, it is often an opportunity to discuss new data before it is submitted for publication in peer-reviewed journals, so it is a chance to obtain feedback on your research. Following a poster presentation at a conference, a study team would continue work to complete any analysis which may not yet have been done or to stimulate interest from funders to conduct additional work in the future.

7.2.2 Submitting an abstract

Most conferences will have an abstract submission period which can be anywhere between 1 and 6 months before the conference. Traditionally, conferences used to take place face-to-face, but now they may take different forms, including hybrid events, in which there may be an option to attend face-to-face or virtually. At some conferences, there is the opportunity to attend virtually in real time and engage with the speakers, e.g. by asking questions. At other conferences, there may be the option to register for the conference but access the content later; this option is usually for a fixed period of time. There are many conferences available at which a researcher can present their data, so it is important to choose the conference carefully to achieve maximum impact. When submitting your abstract to a conference, it is an expectation that the data you present is novel, accurate and has not been published anywhere else. Some conferences will also request information on whether permission has been obtained from all co-authors to submit the work and any other financial disclosures, e.g. commercial, may also be requested.

7.2.3 Designing the poster

Once your abstract has been accepted for publication, it is most likely that you will be asked to present it in the form of a poster. Nowadays, many posters will be presented digitally, but some face-to-face conferences may still give the option to print a poster for presentation at a conference, so it is important to check the requirements for presentation carefully.

7.2.4 General layout

Figure 7.2 provides an example poster layout that could be used for a typical conference presentation, and *Figures 7.3* and *7.4* show actual posters presented at conferences.

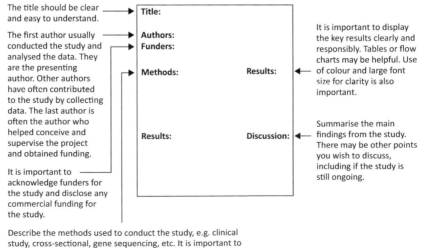

Figure 7.2. Example poster layout.

Below are examples of posters that have been presented at conferences. They are examples of how audits in a clinical setting were used to present data on the use of specific drugs in clinical practice.

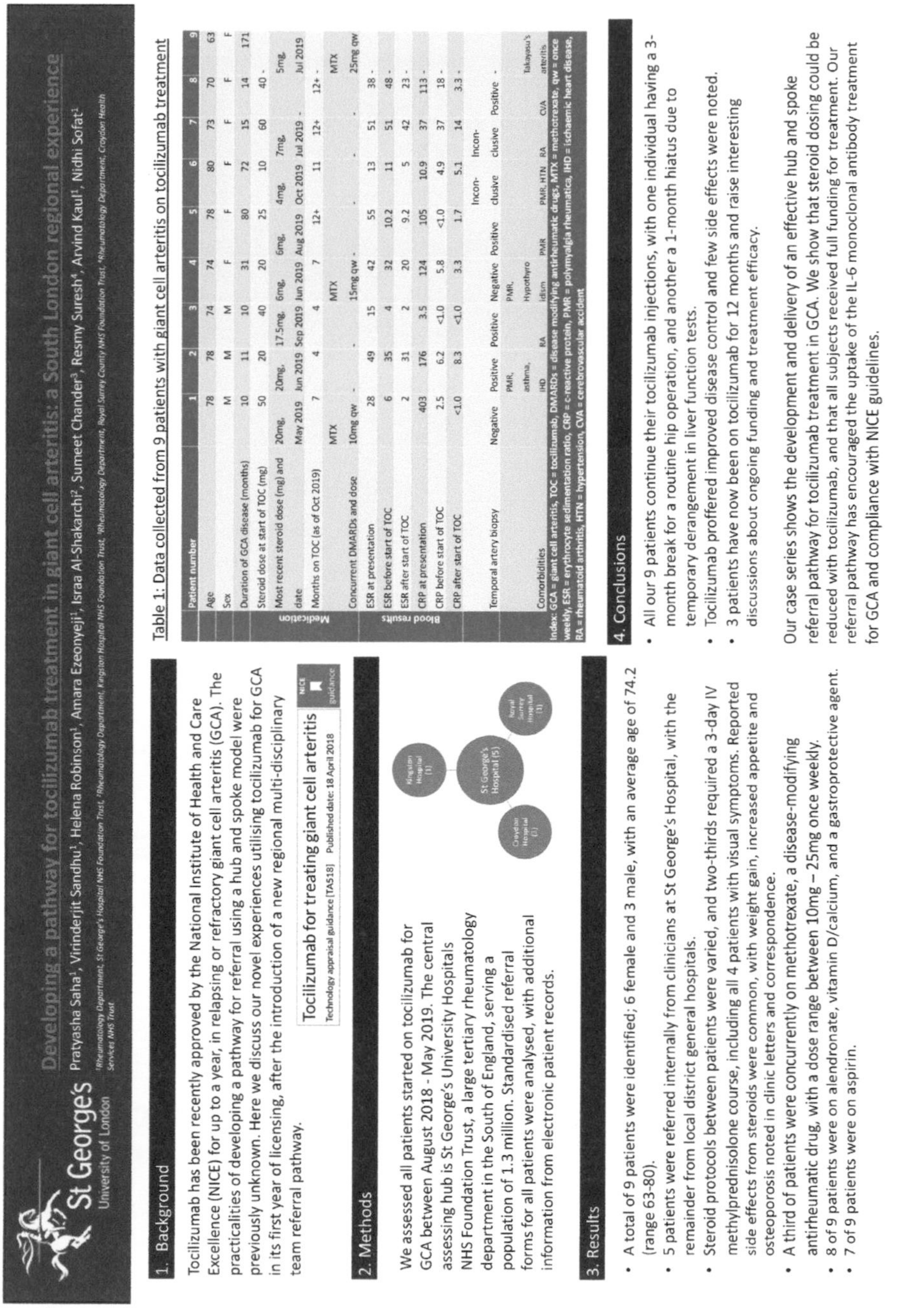

Figure 7.3. Example of a poster presentation.

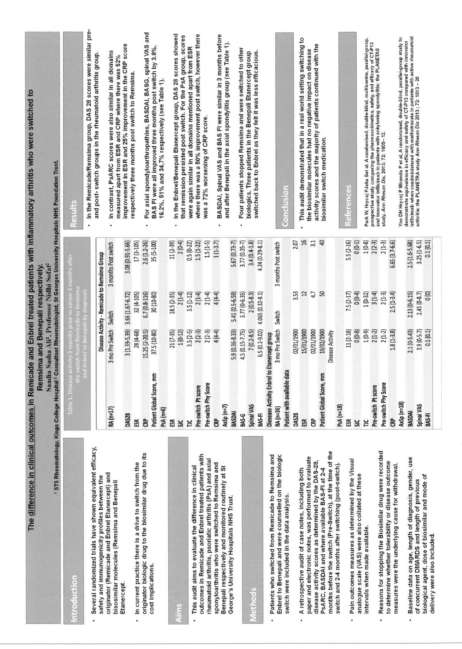

Figure 7.4. Example of a poster presentation.

7.2.5 Presenting the poster

It is important to find out the costs of printing the poster beforehand and if there is a study budget available to cover the costs. Study leave will also need to be arranged. Depending on circumstances, your Institution may assist you with covering study leave costs if there is a study budget that you can apply for.

7.3 Oral presentations

It is often a career highlight for a trainee to present their work as an oral presentation at a conference and there are several guidelines which can be followed to deliver an effective presentation. The general format of the presentation should, similar to the abstract, include the following information: the background to the study; important study methods; a summary of the results; discussion, including future work and acknowledgements; supervisors, funders and collaborators. It is important to check the duration of the presentation, e.g. some may have a stipulated time for presenting, such as 10 minutes, with 5 minutes for questions.

There are several tips for presentation which include designing slides which have a large font size that can be read easily, using bullet points instead of using large amounts of text, using contrasting colours and avoiding the use of distracting special effects. If there is a film or video to play in the presentation, ensure that it works on the platform that is being used for the conference. Ensure that you know who your audience are, e.g. are they medical professionals in the field, trainee doctors, medical students? Is the presentation pitched at the correct level for the audience? It is important to speak confidently, clearly and slowly and avoid using jargon that may not be understood. It is important to practise before presenting and to ensure you stay to time. Many presenters will slow down at the end of the presentation to signpost they have finished speaking and many will end with an acknowledgement slide.

Methods used in the study

- A systematic review was performed of treatments for Covid-19 infection
- Published literature from January 2019 onwards was searched using databases including Medline, PubMed, Embase, Ovid and Cochrane
- A review of all articles in the published literature with the search terms: Covid-19, pharmacological therapies, oxygen was conducted
- All published abstracts identified with these search terms were reviewed to assess for suitability for inclusion in the systematic review

Figure 7.5. Example of a good slide, featuring a large font, bullets to highlight key points, and no special effects. This slide summarises very clearly that a systematic review was performed, the time period for the searches, the key search terms and how they were assessed for suitability in the study.

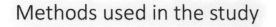

Methods used in the study

- We carried out a systematic review to find out which treatments were published in the literature for the treatment of Covid-19 infection. We performed a literature search of new treatments for Covid-19 infection from journal articles
- Our search was carried out to find literature for new treatments for Covid-19 using a wide variety of databases such as Medline, Pubmed, Embase, Ovid and Cochrane databases
- We used several search terms to retrieve articles from the literature
- After obtaining all the published articles, they were reviewed and checked

Figure 7.6. Example of a poor slide. This slide has unnecessary information with long sentences and an unnecessary tint behind the text. Key information such as the start date for the search and key words that were used to conduct the searches in the systematic review are missing.

7.4   Publications

7.4.1 What type of manuscript?

Once you have completed a piece of research and perhaps also presented it at a conference, it is important to submit your work in peer-reviewed journals for full publication. Having a manuscript accepted for publication allows it to be read more widely by other researchers, the public and policy makers, thereby sharing methodology and results as widely as possible. By adding new findings to the literature, it can help to advance medical knowledge; for example, a clinical trial of a new drug or a new epidemiological study which tracks the course of a disease in a population.

It is important to consider what format your work is likely to take. Full-length research articles are often developed after the completion of a large project, e.g. a clinical study or trial. They often represent several years' work and provide the authors with the opportunity to describe their study methodology and results in some detail. In other cases, another article format may be more suitable, e.g. a letter to the editor about a recent article that has provoked interest, or a case series which may be based on a set of new clinical features in a condition or rare complications. Review articles may be opinion-based pieces, or they could include systematic reviews or meta-analyses in a certain topic area. Further detail on study type selection for specific research questions is provided in *Chapter 2*. A summary of study type and reporting guidelines is shown in *Table 7.2*.

Table 7.2: Summary of study type and reporting characteristics for publishing

Type of study	Considerations in reporting and relevant reporting guidelines
Systematic review and meta-analyses	Study registration in databases, e.g. PROSPERO
	Report study according to guidelines including PRISMA, Cochrane
Randomised controlled trials	Study registration in databases, e.g. clinicaltrials.gov, ISRCTN registry, UKCRC network
	Report study according to guidelines including CONSORT
Cohort studies	Adhere to reporting guidelines in observational study, e.g. STROBE
Case–control studies	Adhere to reporting guidelines in observational study, e.g. STROBE
Cross-sectional studies	Adhere to reporting guidelines in observational study, e.g. STROBE
Case reports	Adhere to guidelines, e.g. CARE, to increase accuracy, transparency and usefulness of case reports

7.4.2 Systematic review and meta-analyses

If you are preparing a systematic review or meta-analysis, you will have conducted your search using guidelines such as Cochrane and PRISMA (see above), which will need reporting according to consensus guidelines. The reviewers of your manuscript will be looking for this information.

7.4.3 Randomised controlled trials

There is a consensus for reporting clinical trials which includes completion of a CONSORT statement which is submitted to the journal. This is to ensure that you can demonstrate that the trial was conducted according to international guidelines. It is also important to report all primary and secondary outcome measures, as was stipulated in the original study protocol and that the authors have not deviated from the original study aims and objectives. For publishing of study protocols, there are SPIRIT guidelines for reporting the necessary information in trial protocols.

7.4.4 Cohort studies

Cohort studies often include large epidemiological datasets which are often reported after several years of assessment and observation. It is important to ensure all the characteristics of the study population are reported and effect sizes are discussed. There are STROBE (Strengthening the Reporting of Observational Studies in Epidemiology) statement guidelines for reporting observational studies. The guidelines recommend standards of reporting in observational studies to strengthen the quality and outcomes of reporting in the literature.

7.4.5 **Case–control studies**

Case–control studies are often conducted with a disease group and compared with healthy control cases. It is important to define the disease and healthy control group clearly with their respective characteristics. Study reporting should also adhere to STROBE guidelines.

7.4.6 **Cross-sectional studies**

In cross-sectional studies, a population is studied for certain characteristics. The researcher can evaluate people at different ages, ethnicities, geographical locations and social backgrounds. Reporting of cases and controls should adhere to the STROBE guidelines in the case of observational cross-sectional studies.

7.4.7 **Case reports**

Case reports may be used to report rare side-effects from a new treatment, or a rare case which has not been seen previously. Such cases are very important to expand knowledge about new treatments in the real-world setting and to raise awareness about rare conditions and their treatment. Case reports should be written according to CARE guidelines (Consensus-based Clinical Case Reporting Guideline Development).

7.4.8 **Authorship**

It is usually expected to include names of authors in the publication who were involved in collecting data, performing experiments, conception and design of the study, data analysis and interpretation. Many journals will request specific contributions from each author to justify authorship.

7.4.9 **Choosing the right journal**

It is important to think carefully about the appropriate journal for submission of work. For example, does the manuscript demonstrate a new treatment paradigm that could lead to a change in clinical practice? If so, then a high impact journal which publishes clinical studies/trials may be the most appropriate for submission, e.g. the *British Medical Journal (BMJ)*, *The Lancet* and the *New England Journal of Medicine (NEJM)*. If the study is in a more specialist area, e.g. the trial of a new surgical technique, then a specialist journal in that field may be more appropriate. It is also useful to read the 'information for authors' sections on specific journal websites to establish specific requirements for journal submission. Information about font, word count, format, reference style and allocation and number of tables and figures is provided by each journal and must be closely adhered to.

Journal **impact factors** may also influence where researchers are likely to submit their manuscript. Impact factors identify how often an article is cited from a particular journal in a given year. Impact factors were originally designed to help librarians in deciding which journals to purchase, but soon afterwards the impact factor became used as a proxy for academic success. The advantage of the journal impact factor system is that it has existed for many years and scientists are experienced with its evaluation. In each specialty area, experience shows that the best journals are those in which it is most difficult to have an article accepted, which are the journals that have a high impact factor. There has been some criticism of journal impact factors over the years. Some researchers have argued that the impact factor may not be a good measure of assessing individual scientific excellence, since there can be a wide variation in citations from article to article within a single journal. Other metrics have developed over the years, e.g. the h-index, to assess author-level metrics. Overall, however, journal impact factors provide a good sense of the leading journals in a specific field and they often publish landmark studies in a particular specialty.

7.4.10 A guide to general format

It is important to spend some time ensuring the formatting of the manuscript is consistent, with sections and sub-headings adhering to the recommendations in the instructions for authors. Good use of English with clarity, conciseness and correctness means that your manuscript is more likely to be understood and will have fewer corrections recommended. It is important to have a clear layout, including double-spacing, adhering to the font size recommended by the journal (usually 12 point) and avoid using jargon. It is important to avoid repetition, ambiguity, exaggeration of results and poor grammar.

The general structure of most manuscripts includes the following sub-headings: Abstract, Introduction, Methods, Results, Discussion, Acknowledgements, References, and Supplementary material. It is important to check specific journal requirements online and adhere to them. Many journals also have a set number of figures or tables which can be submitted. It is important to adhere to journal guidelines to ensure a smooth review process.

7.4.11 The peer review process and revisions

All published manuscripts first have to go through a review process that usually involves at least two experts in the field reviewing the manuscript. Reviewers are provided with criteria against which to review the manuscript, including originality, validity of results, whether the conclusions are appropriate based on the data and whether further statistical analysis is required. Once the manuscript has been written and is ready for submission, it is worth considering if there are any potential peer reviewers who would be well-placed to review your manuscript, based on their expertise and knowledge of the field. Reviewers will often be requested during the online submission process of your manuscript.

Peer-reviewed journals aim to have manuscripts reviewed in a timely manner, e.g. usually within 3–6 weeks, to avoid long delays in publication. Once reviews have been received from reviewers, the journal will make a decision on the article, typically along the following lines:

- 'Accept' with minor revisions. In this instance, the reviewers may comment that the manuscript is generally sound, with some minor edits which need to be addressed, e.g. explaining a figure legend in more detail or adding pertinent references.
- 'Major revisions' recommended followed by further review. In this decision for a manuscript, the reviewers may recommend a new set of experiments are performed, or they may have concerns with the methodology and could ask for new analysis. The authors will usually be given a timeline, e.g. 4–6 weeks, to work on an edited version of the manuscript.
- 'Reject'. This is a disappointing decision to receive from a journal and there may be many reasons for rejection. These include the content of the manuscript not showing enough novelty to be published, issues with the methodology or sample size being too small to prove a biological effect. A journal usually does not allow a manuscript to be resubmitted after a rejection. Authors can continue to work on it to see if it might be more suitable to publish in an alternative journal.

Some submitted manuscripts may be rejected within a very short period of time, especially in cases where the editor is of the view that the article is beyond the scope of the journal, or if there is lack of novelty, or other factors such as small sample size. In the major revisions category, reviewers may request further analysis or experiments. By the examples described, it is important to remember that the peer-review process can be a long one after corrections are submitted back to the journal for reconsideration by the reviewers. The process can take up to six months and sometimes longer. After acceptance for publication, depending on the journal involved, open access charges and other journal charges may need to be paid, so it is important to check details for each journal before submission. In addition, many journals now publish straight after acceptance electronically, but the formal 'paper' publication may follow several months after initial acceptance.

7.5 Evidence-based medicine and implementation science

7.5.1 Evidence-based medicine

The ultimate aim of conducting good research studies is to inform clinical practice and improve patient care. Evidence-based medicine (EBM) refers to the use of the best available research to inform clinical care. EBM can cover many aspects of care, including the accuracy and precision of diagnostic tests, the use of prognostic markers, determining which healthcare strategies provide the best therapeutic, rehabilitative or preventive strategies, and also includes recognition of the patient experience.

In many countries, evidence-based recommendations are developed by independent committees, including professionals and lay members. In a certain condition, e.g.

treatment of hypertension, the available evidence is reviewed by panels and a conclusion reached advising specific treatment recommendations. In many cases, there will be clinical trial evidence from randomised controlled trials, which are considered to be the highest level of evidence. In some cases, meta-analyses may also have been performed on the randomised trials to assess whether a specific drug improves outcomes. In other rarer conditions, randomised controlled trial data may not be available and data such as reports of treatment of smaller groups of participants may be assessed. In the UK, the National Institute for Health and Care Excellence (NICE) publishes evidence-based guidelines on management which are accessible to clinicians and the public (www.nice.org.uk).

7.5.2 Implementation science

There are thousands of research studies carried out worldwide which may have important messages for clinical practice, e.g. implementation of a treatment pathway to improve patient care. However, one of the challenges of clinical research is to assess the validity and outcomes of studies performed, so that effective treatments can be used in clinical care as rapidly and effectively as possible.

Implementation science is the study of methods to promote the uptake of research findings into routine clinical practice so that the quality and effectiveness of health services can be improved. In many conditions, the implementation of a new treatment may take several years to be adopted, due to issues such as infrastructure availability to provide the treatment, funding and treatment pathway development issues.

A recent example of the implementation of a new treatment which was rapidly translated into clinical practice included the results from the RECOVERY trial in the UK, which reported on the use of dexamethasone for the treatment of SARS-CoV-2 infection.

WORKED EXAMPLE
Dexamethasone in hospitalized patients with Covid-19

RECOVERY Collaborative Group (2021) *New Engl J Med*, **384**: 693. doi.org/10.1056/NEJMoa2021436

Background

Covid-19 infection can cause diffuse lung damage. The study team hypothesised that glucocorticoids might modulate the lung injury caused by inflammation in people with Covid-19 infection. If the treatment with dexamethasone was effective, it may reduce the progression to respiratory failure and death.

The RECOVERY study group, which included numerous hospital sites across the UK, carried out a controlled, open-label trial in which participants who were in hospital with Covid-19 infection were offered a range of different treatments which included dexamethasone.

Results

The authors evaluated a total of 2104 participants who were randomised to receive dexamethasone and 4321 who received usual care. The analysis showed that 482 subjects (22.9%) in the dexamethasone group and 1110 patients (25.7%) in the usual-care group died within 28 days of randomisation (age-adjusted rate ratio, 0.83; 95% confidence interval, 0.75–0.93; P <0.001). Interestingly, the incidence of death was lower than that in the usual-care group in participants receiving invasive mechanical ventilation (29.3% versus 41.4%).

Comments

Implications of RECOVERY trial with dexamethasone:

- The RECOVERY trial was set up very early on during the Covid-19 pandemic, which meant that study data was collected early in the disease outbreak on a UK-wide level, which increased the power of the study and allowed early reporting of results.
- Regulatory authorities were able to rapidly evaluate data submitted to assess the outcomes of the trials conducted, which led to rapid licensing of drugs within a few months; a process which hitherto usually took several years.
- As a consequence of the convincing results from the RECOVERY trial, the use of dexamethasone became widely adopted into clinical guidelines, including the NICE guidelines in the UK (www.nice.org.uk/guidance/ng191) and international guidelines, such as those issued by the National Institutes of Health (NIH) in the USA (www.covid19treatmentguidelines.nih.gov/about-the-guidelines/whats-new).
- As a consequence of the use of dexamethasone in the RECOVERY trial, other immunomodulatory drugs were also tested, including tocilizumab and baricitinib, both of which are now also licensed for the management of patients hospitalised with Covid-19.

7.6   Chapter summary

Presenting and publishing research is often a highlight of a research project, when the research team have the opportunity to present their data to a wider audience, including the research community, funders, commissioners and the public. Medical writing has several guidelines and recommendations for publishing which need to be adhered to. Due consideration of the issues highlighted in this chapter will enable the researcher to publish their work and ensure that it creates an impactful addition to existing literature in the field.

7.7 References and further reading

https://arc-sl.nihr.ac.uk/research-and-implementation/our-research-methods/implementation-science: this website discusses implementation science, which is the study of methods and strategies to take up interventions that have been found to be effective into routine clinical practice.

ClinicalTrials.gov: this website contains a database of privately and publicly funded clinical studies from around the world. It contains information about clinical trials recruiting participants with particular conditions and which countries are involved. Reports of data from the trial are also posted on the website once it is available.

www.consort-statement.org: CONSORT stands for the Consolidated Standards of Reporting Trials and encompasses various initiatives developed by the CONSORT group to address standards that should be adhered to in reporting randomised controlled trials.

https://ebm.bmj.com: this website hosts the *BMJ* journal entitled *BMJ Evidence-Based Medicine*. It focuses on tools, methods and concepts that are important in practising evidence-based medicine and delivering impactful and trustworthy evidence.

www.equator-network.org/reporting-guidelines/spirit-2013-statement-defining-standard-protocol-items-for-clinical-trials: the SPIRIT guidelines for reporting study protocols are described.

www.equator-network.org/reporting-guidelines/strobe: this equator network website contains information about the various reporting guidelines for observational studies, including CONSORT (randomised trials), STROBE (observational studies), PRISMA (systematic reviews), SPIRIT (study protocols), STARD (diagnostic/prognostic studies), CARE (case reports) and AGREE (clinical practice guidelines).

www.nihr.ac.uk/documents/nihr-policy-on-clinical-trial-registration-and-disclosure-of-results/12252: this website discusses the NIHR policy on timely disclosure of results, which are critical to ensure full transparency of clinical trials funded by NIHR.

Turabian, K.L. (2020) *A Manual for Writers of Research Papers, Theses, and Dissertations*, 9th edition. The University of Chicago Press.

Glossary

Absolute risk reduction (ARR) – the relative risk in the intervention group minus the relative risk in the control group.

Adverse event (AE) – any unintended or untoward response in a study participant to whom an investigational medicinal product (IMP) has been administered.

Adverse reaction (AR) – unintended or untoward reactions in study participants to IMPs or interventions. ARs differ from AEs in that there is at least a reasonable possibility that the reaction is due to the IMP.

Alpha value – the probability of type I error or the threshold for statistical significance.

Alternative hypothesis – the hypothesis that there is a difference in the outcome of interest between groups.

Arms – the specific groups or subgroups in a study that receive a particular intervention (or no intervention) according to the study protocol.

Audit trails – records of the data collection process and rationale behind the decisions made throughout the study.

Beta value – the probability of a type II error.

Bias – a systematic difference between the results from a study and the true data.

Blinding – the method whereby doctors, researchers and patients are not aware of the treatment (or no treatment) group the subjects are in, so that they cannot influence the conduct or results of the study.

Case report form (CRF) – a paper form, usually in the format of a questionnaire, used to collect information from each participant.

Chief investigator (CI) – an individual who takes the overall lead for the research project.

Coding – a way of organising data in a structured manner by breaking down the data into categories and then assigning labels to these.

Collaboration – public and patient involvement in which researchers and members of the public jointly design, carry out or disseminate research in an equal partnership.

Computer-assisted qualitative data analysis software (CAQDAS) – software which can aid with qualitative data analysis, such as speeding up transcription or storing codes.

Confidence interval (CI) – the range of values in which there is a specified probability that the value of a parameter lies. Most commonly, the 95% confidence interval is used.

Confounding – a confounding variable affects the independent and the dependent variable. When confounding is present, spurious conclusions can be made regarding the relationship between the dependent and independent variable.

Constructivist position – explains behaviour through individuals' own subjective world view.

Consultation – public and patient involvement in which patients or members of the public attend meetings to share their views, in order to inform research decisions.

Content analysis – qualitative research analysis strategies which use a systematic coding and categorising approach to find themes within a dataset.

Convenience sampling – involves all people who happen to be most accessible to the investigator. Convenience sampling is a quick and inexpensive technique for selecting sample participants.

Data saturation – the point at which no new concepts emerge from the data.

Deductive – top-down approach to analysing qualitative data. The researcher begins with a set of predetermined codes and then finds excerpts to fit those codes.

Degrees of freedom (df) – the sample size minus the number of parameters that have to be estimated to calculate the statistic.

Delegation log – this summarises the individual members of the site team and identifies which members are delegated to perform different tasks.

Dependent variable – a variable that is measured whose value depends on the value of the independent variable. The dependent variable is predicted by the explanatory variable in regression analyses.

Discourse analysis – a qualitative research analysis approach which focuses on linguistic analysis of the flow of communication within its social, cultural or political context.

Epistemology – a branch of philosophy that studies the nature of knowledge.

Explanatory variable – a variable whose value predicts the value of the dependent variable in a regression analysis.

Face validity – whether the test appears (at face value) to measure what it claims to.

Field notes – notes recorded throughout an interview. These include reflections on the interview, the environment and body language of the participant.

Fixed effects model – a statistical regression model in which the intercept of the regression model is allowed to vary freely across individuals or groups. The model is often used in data to control for individual-specific attributes.

Forest plot – a graphical display of estimated results from several scientific studies that have addressed the same question, along with the overall result by combining data from all the studies.

Funnel plot – a graphical representation of the size of trials plotted against the effect size that they are reporting.

Grounded theory – a qualitative research analysis approach which develops theories based on the iterative collection of data.

Hazard ratio – a ratio of the hazard rates in two different groups.

Impact factor – the impact factor of an academic journal is an index calculated by Clarivate that reflects the annual mean number of citations of articles published in a given journal that is indexed by Clarivate's Web of Science.

Incidence – refers to the number of individuals who develop a specific disease or experience a specific health-related event during a specific time period, e.g. a month or year.

Independent variable – a variable whose value affects the value of the dependent variable.

Inductive – bottom-up approach to qualitative analysis where the researcher derives codes from the data.

Informed consent – the process whereby a healthcare provider educates a patient or a study participant about the risks, benefits or alternatives of a given procedure or intervention.

Internal validity – researchers seek to ensure that a study measures or tests what is actually intended.

Interpretative phenomenological analysis (IPA) – a qualitative research analysis method which aims to understand how subjects experience the world within a particular context (phenomenon).

Iterative – an approach to research where the methodology or analysis are refined based on what has been found so far.

Likelihood ratio (LR) – the likelihood of a test result in patients with the disease divided by the likelihood of a test result in patients without the disease.

Memo – notes which explain thought patterns throughout data analysis when using grounded theory.

Moderator – someone who is responsible for guiding the discussion during a focus group. They must ensure the discussion stays on topic and that everyone has an equal chance to speak.

Narrative analysis – a qualitative research analysis method which aims to understand how people construct stories and narratives from personal experiences.

Negative predictive value – the proportion of individuals with a negative test who do not have the disease.

Normal distribution – a symmetrical distribution that follows a bell-shaped curve with a single peak. Mathematically, the normal distribution follows a Gaussian curve and is symmetrical around the mean value.

Null hypothesis – a hypothesis that states there is no difference in the outcome of interest between the defined groups.

Number needed to treat (NNT) – the number of patients needed to treat in order to prevent one additional adverse outcome.

Odds ratio – the odds of an outcome in the exposed group divided by the odds of the outcome in the unexposed group.

Ontology – a branch of philosophy that studies the nature of reality.

P **value** – the probability of obtaining the result, or something more extreme, if the null hypothesis is true.

Parametric tests – tests that are based on assumptions about the population from which the sample was taken. In order to use parametric statistics, the population distribution frequency should follow a normal distribution and the variances in each group should be equal.

Patient and public engagement (PPE) – informing the patients or public about research findings.

Patient and public involvement (PPI) – researchers working in active partnership with patients and the public to carry out research.

Patient information leaflet (PIL) – written information given to potential subjects of a clinical trial. It summarises all information about the clinical trial relevant to the participants' involvement.

Positive predictive value – the proportion of individuals with a positive test who have the disease.

Positivist position – method of analysis that uses empirical scientific measurement to understand the social and material world.

Prevalence – the proportion of a population who have a specific characteristic in a given time period.

Principal investigator (PI) – an individual who takes responsibility for the conduct of research at a study site.

Prolonged engagement – the researcher spending time immersed in an environment to understand the context and culture of the person and situation being investigated.

Publication bias – a type of bias that occurs when the outcome of the study biases the decision to publish or not.

Purposive sampling – a type of non-probability sampling where the researchers use their own judgement to choose participants with certain demographics to invite to their study.

Quota sampling – non-probability sampling where researchers decide on quotas to fill based on certain characteristics.

Random effects model – this is a statistical model where the model parameters are random variables.

Random sampling – every person in a population has an equal chance to be selected in research. A complete population is needed in the sampling frame. Different tools such as a random number generator can be used.

Recall bias – systematic error that occurs when study participants incorrectly remember events or experiences.

Reflexivity – the researcher acknowledging the influence of their experiences, assumptions and beliefs on the research process.

Relative risk – the risk of an outcome in the exposed group divided by the risk of an outcome in the unexposed group.

Respondent validation – asking the participant to verify that the interview transcript is accurate and that the interpretation resonates with their experience.

Reverse causality – this means that X and Y are associated, but not in the way that would be expected. For example, instead of X causing a change in Y, it is the other way around, i.e. Y causing a change in X. In epidemiology, reverse causality is when the exposure–disease process is reversed, i.e. the exposure causes the risk factor.

Sampling methods – the process of how and which research parameters are used to collect samples from a test population.

Selection bias – systematic error that occurs when the characteristics of study participants differ systematically from the population of interest.

Sensitivity – the proportion of individuals without the disease who test negative using the test.

Snowball sampling – asking participants to recommend other people they know to be recruited to the study.

Specificity – the proportion of individuals with the disease who test positive using the test.

Standard deviation (SD) – a commonly reported measure of spread that quantifies how much dataset values differ from the sample mean. Mathematically, the standard deviation is equal to the square root of the variance.

Standard error of the mean (SEM) – a measure of the difference between the sample estimate and the population parameter. The SEM quantifies the precision of the sample estimate.

Statistical power – the probability of rejecting the null hypothesis when it is false. It is defined mathematically as 1 – beta.

Statistically significant – means that a result is unlikely to be due to chance. Researchers often use the P value to express the probability of obtaining a difference from a tested set of samples.

Stratified sampling – if a population has mixed characteristics, every character needs to be proportionate so that it represents a sample. A large population can be divided into small subgroups based on relevant characteristics.

Study sponsor – an organisation or partnership responsible for the initiation, management and financing of a clinical study.

***t* distribution** – a widely used probability distribution in statistics. The shape of the t distribution is similar to the normal distribution, characterised by its degrees of freedom.

Thematic analysis – a qualitative research analysis method which identifies, analyses and interprets patterns or themes within a dataset.

Theme – in thematic analysis a theme captures something important about how the data relates to the research question.

Topic guide – has a list of the main topics and questions and is used in an interview to guide the discussion and maintain consistency across interviews.

Triangulation – identifying convergences of data obtained via using multiple methods or datasets to address a research question.

***T*-score** – the relationship of the mean of the dataset to the mean of the population. Used in preference to the Z-score when the sample size is small.

Type I error – a false positive result. This occurs when a significant difference between groups is reported when in reality, one does not exist.

Type II error – a false negative result. This occurs when it is incorrectly reported that there is no difference between the two groups when in reality, one exists.

User-led research – research that is managed and directed by patients or members of the public.

Validity – assessment of whether the project is credible. The research is aimed to be transferable, dependable and the findings can be confirmed.

Variance – a commonly used measure of spread equal to the squared standard deviation.

Z-score – the relationship of the mean of the dataset to the mean of the population.

Index

Bold indicates main entry